the**facts**

Ankylosing Spondylitis and Axial Spondyloarthritis

also available in the facts series

the**facts**

Ankylosing Spondylitis and Axial Spondyloarthritis

SECOND EDITION

MUHAMMAD ASIM KHAN, MD, FRCP, MACP, MACR

Professor Emeritus of Medicine,
Case Western Reserve University,
Cleveland, Ohio, USA

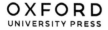
OXFORD
UNIVERSITY PRESS

Great Clarendon Street, Oxford, OX2 6DP,
United Kingdom

Oxford University Press is a department of the University of Oxford.
It furthers the University's objective of excellence in research, scholarship,
and education by publishing worldwide. Oxford is a registered trade mark of
Oxford University Press in the UK and in certain other countries

First Edition published in 2002
Second Edition published in 2023
Impression: 1

Published in the United States of America by Oxford University Press
198 Madison Avenue, New York, NY 10016, United States of America

British Library Cataloguing in Publication Data

Data available

Library of Congress Control Number: 2022938866

ISBN 978–0–19–886415–8

DOI: 10.1093/oso/9780198864158.001.0001

Printed and bound by
CPI Group (UK) Ltd, Croydon, CR0 4YY

Dedication

I dedicate this book to my father, Umar Khan, my mother, Hameeda Khanam, and to her father, Sadr-ud-Din Khan (a high school principal who retired as inspector of schools) for having inculcated in me the passion to pursue knowledge and impart it to others. They all worked tirelessly to re-establish when we became refugees, uprooted from our ancestral lands when I was a little over three years old. Therefore, I also dedicate this book to all the refugees like me in this world who may still be longing for a home, and most of them also happen to share my faith.

Advance praise

'Written for patients by a patient who is also a leading authority on spondyloarthritis, this book is an essential reference and reading for people living with axial spondyloarthritis—with ankylosing spondylitis as its prototype—and their caregivers who want to learn about the disease and how to manage it well.'

Michael Mallinson,
Patient Advocate and Volunteer,
Axial Spondyloarthritis International Federation (ASIF)

Preface

There have been tremendous advances in clinical understanding, early disease recognition, and more effective management of ankylosing spondylitis (AS) and related diseases. The advent of newer imaging methods, such as magnetic resonance imaging (MRI) and very low-dose computerized tomography (CT), have also facilitated early diagnosis and initiation of increasingly more effective (but costly) drugs called "biologics" (administered by injection under the skin or by intravenous infusion), and most recently JAK-inhibitors that are taken orally as tablets. These drugs target inflammatory proteins (cytokines), such as tumor necrosis factor (TNF) and interleukin-17 (IL-17).

All these new development and progress in diagnosis and management of AS and related diseases has necessitated this second edition of the book. I have updated its title by adding the term "Axial Spondyloarthritis" that requires some explanation.

The term "spondyloarthritis" (or SpA) refers to a family of chronic inflammatory non-contagious (non-infectious) forms of arthritis involving the spine and the limbs that share many of their clinical features and genetic predisposing factors. Those patients with SpA who primarily have inflammation of the joints and ligaments of the back and neck (i.e., the axial skeleton) are now sub-classified as having "axial spondyloarthritis" (axSpA); whereas those with involvement predominantly of the peripheral (distal) limb joints (other than hip and shoulder joints that are part of the axial skeleton), are labeled as having "peripheral SpA." The typical example of axSpA is AS, while that of peripheral SpA is psoriatic arthritis (PsA).

X-ray evidence of damage to the sacroiliac joints (sacroiliitis) is required for the diagnosis of AS. We first reported in 1985 that one can clinically recognize the disease even when there is no X-ray evidence of sacroiliitis. We called it "spondylitic disease without radiological evidence of sacroiliitis." It is now called "non-radiographic axSpA" (nr-axSpA). The name axSpA encompasses both nr-axSpA and AS.

Most of the current knowledge about axSpA was gained when the disease was called AS, and this is my reason for the use of both AS and axSpA in the title of this second edition. It is my hope that the third edition of this book will simply be titled *Axial Spondyloarthritis: The Facts*. The term "radiographic axSpA" (r-axSpA) has sometimes been equated with AS but I have preferred to use the term AS in this book as it is the most widely accepted name.

This book is written in a clear and accessible style with American English spellings for patients and their families and friends. But it is also ideal for students and healthcare professionals of all levels who are looking for concise and practical information on all aspects of AS/axSpA. Discussions about the associated forms of SpA, including PsA, reactive arthritis, inflammatory bowel disease associated SpA, juvenile SpA, and some other diseases that may be confused with SpA (the so-called disease mimickers or look-alikes) are also discussed. A glossary of medical terms, a list of abbreviations, links to patient support groups and other helpful organizations, a list of medical references for further reading, and an index are also included.

People who are knowledgeable about their disease show more self-responsibility, comply better with recommended treatment, and are more likely to make positive behavioral changes that will help them achieve an improved health status in the long run. I hope this book will serve people living with AS/axSpA and their families and friends in their need for self-education.

Lastly, I would add that this book provides a general information that cannot replace the care and knowledge provided by your professional healthcare providers. You need to consult them if you have questions as you read this book.

Muhammad Asim Khan
Professor Emeritus of Medicine
Case Western Reserve University, Cleveland, Ohio, USA

Acknowledgments

I am most grateful to my wife Mastoora and my sons Ali and Raza for their help; and also very thankful to the many patients, colleagues, and students who have, over the years, enhanced my knowledge of ankylosing spondylitis, an illness I have myself lived with for more than sixty-six years.

Contents

Abbreviations

3D	three-dimensional
AAU	acute anterior uveitis
ACE	angiotensin-converting-enzyme
ACR	American College of Rheumatology
ADL	activities of daily living
AI	artificial intelligence
AS	ankylosing spondylitis
ASAS	Assessment of SpondyloArthritis international Society
ASAS HI	ASAS Health Index
ASDAS	Ankylosing Spondylitis Disease Activity Score
ASDAS_CRP	Ankylosing Spondylitis Disease Activity Score based on CRP
ASIF	Axial Spondyloarthritis International Federation
ASQoL	ankylosing spondylitis quality of life measure
AP	anteroposterior
axSpA	axial spondyloarthritis
BASDAI	Bath Ankylosing Spondylitis Disease Activity Index
BASFI	Bath Ankylosing Spondylitis Functional Index
BAS-G	Bath Ankylosing Spondylitis Patient Global score
BASMI	Bath Ankylosing Spondylitis Metrology Index
BASRI	Bath Ankylosing Spondylitis Radiology Index
b-DMARD	biologic DMARD
BiPAP	bilevel positive airways pressure
BMC	bone mineral content
BMD	bone mineral density
BMI	body mass index
CASPAR	Classification Criteria for Psoriatic Arthritis
CBD	cannabidiol
CD	Crohn's disease

CDC	Centers for Disease Control and Prevention in the United States.
c-DMARD	conventional DMARD
CD-SpA	CD-associated spondyloarthritis
CES-D	Center for Epidemiological Studies Depression
CLBP	chronic low back pain
CNO	chronic non-infectious osteitis
COA	Certificate of Analysis
COX	cyclooxygenase
CPAP	continuous positive airway pressure
CRP	C-reactive protein
cs-DMARD	conventional synthetic DMARD
CT	computed tomography
DAS	disease activity score
DEXA (or DXA)	dual energy x-ray absorptiometry
DISH	diffuse idiopathic skeletal hyperostosis
DKK	abbreviation for protein named Dickkopf
DMARD	disease modifying anti-rheumatic drug
DXA	dual-energy X-ray absorptiometry
EAM	extra articular manifestation
EMA	Europeans Medicines Agency
EMAS	European Mapping of Axial Spondyloarthritis
EMR	electronic medical record
ERAP	endoplasmic reticulum aminopeptidase
ESR	erythrocyte sedimentation rate
ESSG	European Spondyloarthropathy Study Group criteria
EULAR	European Alliance of Associations for Rheumatology
FACIT	Functional Assessment of Chronic Illness Therapy
FDA	Food and Drug Administration of USA
GI	gastrointestinal
GP	general practitioner
GWAS	gnome-wide association study
HAQ	Health Assessments Questionnaire
HAQ-DI	HAQ Disability Index
HAQ-S	HAQ spondylitis
HCP	healthcare providers
HLA	human leucocyte antigen
HR-QoL	health-related quality of life
IASP	International Association for the Study of Pain

IBD	inflammatory bowel disease
IBP	inflammatory back pain
Ig	immunoglobulin
IL	Interleukin, such as IL-17 and IL-23
IBS	irritable bowel syndrome
JAK	Janus kinase
JAKi	Janus kinase inhibitor
JAKin	JAK inhibitors
JAS	juvenile AS
JIA	juvenile idiopathic arthritis
MCS	Mental Component Score
MFI	Multidimensional Fatigue Inventory
MHC	major histocompatibility complex
mNY	modified New York (criteria for ankylosing spondylitis)
MRI	magnetic resonance imaging
mSASSS	modified Stoke Ankylosing Spondylitis Spine Score
NASS	National Axial Spondyloarthritis Society
NHANES	National Health and Nutritional Examination Survey
NHS	National Health Service of UK
NIH	National Institute of Health of USA
nr-axSpA	non-radiographic axial spondyloarthritis
NSAID	nonsteroidal anti-inflammatory drugs
OA	osteoarthritis
OCT	optical coherence tomography
OTC	over-the-counter
PAMP	pathogen-associated molecular pattern
PASS	Patient-Acceptable Symptom State
PCP	primary healthcare provider
PCS	Physical Component Score
PD	phosphodiesterase
PET	positron emission tomography
PGA	Patient Global Assessment
PGE2	prostaglandin E2
PhD	Doctor of Philosophy
PPD	purified protein derivative
PPR	pattern recognition receptor
PRO	Patient Reported Outcome
PROM	Patient Reported Outcome Measure

PsA	psoriatic arthritis
QoL	quality of life
RA	rheumatoid arthritis
RAPID3	Routine Assessment of Patient Index Data 3
r-axSpA	radiographic axSpA
RCT	randomized controlled trial
SAARD	slow-acting anti-rheumatic drug
SAPHO	synovitis, acne, palmoplantar pustulosis, hyperostosis, and aseptic osteomyelitis
SASSS	Stoke Ankylosing Spondylitis Spine Score
SEA	seronegative enthesitis and arthritis
SF-36	Short-Study Form-36
SI	sacroiliac (or sacroiliitis)
SI joint or SIJ	sacroiliac joint
SpA	spondyloarthritis or spondyloarthropathy
THA	total hip arthroplasty
THC	tetrahydrocannabinol
THR	total hip joint replacement
TMJ	temporo-mandibular joint
TNF	tumor necrosis factor
TNFi	tumor necrosis factor inhibitor
ts-DMARDs	targeted synthetic-DMARDs
UC	ulcerative colitis
VAS	visual analog scale
WBC	white blood-cell count
WHO	World Health Organization
WLQ-25	Work Limitations Questionnaire-25
WPAI	Work Productivity and Activity Impairment

1

What is ankylosing spondylitis?

 Key points

- Ankylosing spondylitis (AS) is a chronic (long-term), slowly progressive, and painful inflammatory arthritis of the sacroiliac (SI) joints and the spine that can lead to gradually progressive impairment of spinal mobility.

- It affects both males and females, and the symptoms typically start during adolescence and early adulthood, and it is very uncommon for the symptoms to begin after age 45.

- The inflammation can also involve the hip and shoulder joints, and less often other limb joints, such as knees, ankles, and heels.

- One or more episodes of acute eye inflammation (acute anterior uveitis) can occur in >30% of patients, and 6 to 10% suffer from psoriasis and/or inflammatory bowel disease.

- The disease is observed worldwide with very variable prevalence, e.g., it affects one in 200 (0.5% prevalence) adults of European ancestry, but is very uncommon in most of the sub-Saharan African populations.

- Its cause is not fully understood but is largely genetically determined, and there is a strong association with a gene called *HLA-B27*.

- There is no cure as yet but most patients can be very well managed if diagnosed and treated early with increasingly effective, though costly, drugs that markedly reduce the risk of irreversible structural damage and help patients pursue a very active and productive lifestyle.

Ankylosing Spondylitis and Axial Spondyloarthritis, Second Edition. Muhammad Asim Khan, Oxford University Press.
© Oxford University Press 2023. DOI: 10.1093/oso/9780198864158.003.0001

Introduction

Ankylosing spondylitis (AS) is a chronic (progressive) painful inflammatory rheumatic non-contagious (non-infectious) disease that involves the back, i.e. the sacroiliac (SI) joints and the spine, that often results in some degree of stiffness (decreased flexibility) of the spine (Figure 1.1). The word *ankylosing* comes from the Greek root *ankylos*, meaning bent, although it has now come to imply something that restricts motion (stiffening) and may ultimately result in fusion. When the joint loses its mobility and becomes stiff it is said to be anky-losed. The word *spondylitis* means inflammation in the joints of the spine, and is derived from *spondylos*, which is the Greek word for vertebra, and *-itis*, which implies presence of inflammation. The name therefore suggests that AS is an inflammatory disease of the spine that can lead to stiffening of the back. It is important to point out that the words spondylitis and spondyloarthritis should not be confused with *spondylosis*, which relates to wear and tear in the spinal column (degenerative disc disease) as we get older.

Ankylosing spondylitis in history

Skeletal specimens in several museum collections testify to the existence of AS from the earliest times. But its first definite anatomical description can be credited to Bernard Conner (1666–1698). He was an Irish physician studying medicine in France when some farmers brought him a skeleton they had found in a cemetery. He wrote in his report, accompanied by the drawing of the skeleton (see Figure 1.2), that the bones were "so straightly and intimately joined, their ligaments perfectly bony, and their articulations so effaced, that they really made but one uniform continuous bone."

The clinical descriptions of the disease date from the late nineteenth cen-tury, with a series of publications in the 1890s by Vladimir von Bechterew (1857–1927) in St Petersburg, Russia, Pierre Marie (1853–1940) in France, and Adolf Strümpell (1853–1926) in Germany. Report of the earliest X-ray examination of a patient with AS was published in 1899, and the characteristic X-ray finding of obliteration of the SI joints was described in 1934.

The name ankylosing spondylitis is widely in use in English speaking countries, with its translation *spondylarthrite ankylosante* in French, *spondylitis ankylopoëtica* in Dutch, and *espondilartritis ankylosante* in Spanish. Older names include *Morbus Bechterew* (Bekhterew's or Bekhterev's disease), *Bekhterev-Strümpell-Marie disease* and *Marie-Strümpell spondylitis*. Although the use of eponyms is now discouraged for naming a disease, the term: "Morbus Bechterew" is still being widely used in German-speaking countries. Other names that have been used include *spondyloarthritis ankylopoëtica, pelvospondylitis ossificans*, and

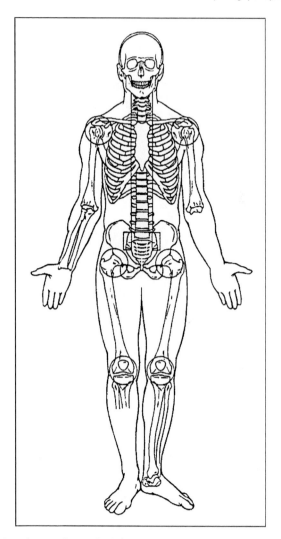

Figure 1.1 Sites that may be involved in AS. The most involved sites are the sacroiliac joints and the spine. They are marked by rectangles. Other, relatively less commonly involved sites are hip and shoulder joints, and less often the knee joints. These sites are marked by circles.

Reproduced with permission from Khan MA. "Spondyloarthropathies" in Hunder G (ed), *Atlas of Rheumatology.* Philadelphia, PA: Current Medicine Philadelphia, 2005, 151–80.

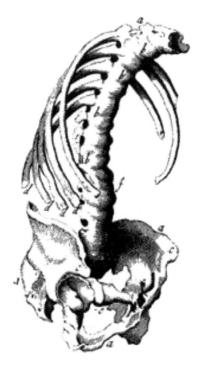

Figure 1.2 First representation of a skeleton with AS in its final state by Bernard Conner, London, 1695.

the laymmen's terms *bamboo spine* and *poker back*. In the US the disease was wrongly called "*rheumatoid spondylitis*" up until early 1960s because of a mistaken belief that it was just a variant of rheumatoid arthritis (RA).

Structure of the spine

The spine, also called the spinal or vertebral column or the backbone, consists of 24 vertebrae that are stacked one above the other, separated from each other by intervertebral discs that act as shock absorbers during mechanical stress, and are held together by strong ligaments and 110 small joints. The spinal column is shown in lateral and front views in Figure 1.3, divided into three main sections:

- *the upper part* (the neck or cervical spine) has 7 vertebrae and is the most mobile part of the spine.

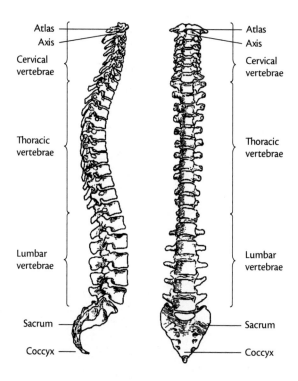

Figure 1.3 The vertebral (spinal) column.

◆ *the middle part* (thoracic spine) has 12 vertebrae, and each has a rib attached to the vertebra on either side by two joints called costo-vertebral and costo-transverse joints. The 12 ribs on either side make up the chest wall, and they are attached in the front to the breastbone (sternum) by costo-chondral junctions. The term *costo* stands for the rib and *chondral* stands for cartilage.

◆ *the lower part* (lumbar spine) has 5 vertebrae, the lowermost (5th) lumbar vertebra sits on a bone called the sacrum.

What is the sacroiliac joint?

The sacrum bone looks like a keystone in the circular bony pelvis formed together with the right and left pelvic bones. It is attached on either side to ilium (the major part of the pelvic bone) by joints called the *sacroiliac* (SI) joints (Figure 1.4). The inflammation usually starts first at these two joints in patients

5

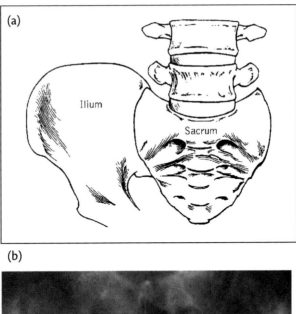

(a)

Ilium

Sacrum

(b)

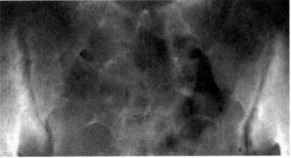

Figure 1.4 The sacroiliac joint: (a) location of the right sacroiliac joint marked by the line separating the sacrum from the ilium, as viewed from the front; (b) pelvic X-ray showing irregularities (bony erosions) of both right and left sacroiliac joints, a characteristic feature of AS.

(b) Reproduced with permission from Khan MA. "Spondyloarthropathies" in Hunder G (ed), *Atlas of Rheumatology.* Philadelphia, PA: Current Medicine Philadelphia, 2005, 151–80.

with AS. Figure 1.5 shows a simplified sketch as viewed from inside the pelvis of a removed left pelvic bone. The darker area depicts the site for attachment of ligamentous and the lighter area (shaped like a boomerang) represents its "synovial" part. The adjacent lower-back part of the pelvic bone that bears our weight when we are sitting down is called the *ischium* or the gluteal tuberosity (cushioned by the overlying buttock muscles) of the pelvic bone. The front part

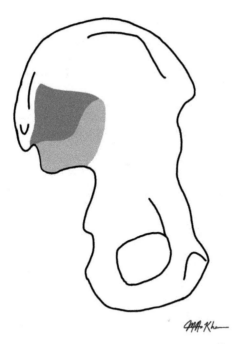

Figure 1.5 The sacroiliac joint area, as visualized from the inner side of the separated left pelvic bone, is shown in two shades of gray; the darker area depicts the ligamentous part and the lighter area (shaped like a boomerang) forms its "synovial" part. Just behind the ligamentous part is the area called the ischium (or the gluteal tuberosity) that bears our weight when we are sitting down. The front lower part of the pelvic bone is called the pubis that forms a junction (called the pubic junction or pubic symphysis) with the other pelvic bone.

of the pelvic bone is called the *pubis* that joins with its counterpart from the other side to form the pubic junction (or *pubic symphysis*).

What is the axial skeleton?

The axial skeleton includes the SI joints, the spine (including the neck), the "root joints" of the limbs (hip and shoulder joints), all the joints and ligamentous structures in the spine, the attachment of the ribs to the back and to the breastbone in the front, as well as attachment of the collar bones *(clavicles)* to the shoulder girdles (by *acromioclavicular joints*) and the *breast-bone* (by *manubrioclavicular joints*). The sites of attachments of the ribs to the breastbone are called *costochondral junctions*. These sites can be involved in AS, and so can the junction between the two parts (*manubrium* and *sternum*) of the breastbone.

The disease symptoms and severity vary from person to person. The disease in some patients may be relatively mild or stay limited to the SI joints and the lumbar spine.

Chronic inflammatory back pain and stiffness

Symptoms typically start during the third decade of life (with a wide age range from 12 to 45), with the mean age of about 24 years (even younger in some of the developing parts of the world). The leading initial symptom is chronic (lasting for more than 3 months) low back pain and stiffness of gradual (insidious) onset that results from inflammation of the SI joints and the lumbar spine. It can initially be felt in the lower back or buttocks area and some patients may complain that their pain initially alternated from one side to the other (alternating buttock pain). The pain may also be felt down the upper part of the back of the thigh but it does not radiate all the way down the lower legs.

The pain and stiffness get worse with prolonged physical inactivity and rest, especially at late hours of the night and early morning. They persist for more than half an hour after waking up, and they ease up after taking a hot shower, walking around, or exercising, *but not with rest*. To remember the 5 salient features of inflammatory back pain (IBP) we have proposed a mnemonic—"IPAIN"—that makes it easier to remember (Box 1.1). It is unlike the common (ubiquitous) back pain or sprain, often called mechanical or non-specific back pain.

Box 1.1 IPAIN: a mnemonic for inflammatory back pain

IPAIN
Insidious onset
Pain at night (with improvement upon getting up)
Age at onset <45 years
Improvement with exercise
No improvement with rest

Reproduced with permission from Ozgocmen S, Akgul O, Khan MA. "Mnemonic for assessment of the spondyloarthritis international society criteria" *J Rheumatol*. 2010 Sep;37(9):1978.

Some people may complain of only transient episodes of lower-back pain with remission periods in between before their symptoms become persistent. In others, the first symptoms may not be in the back, but they may complain of painful heels and limb joints, especially hip and/or shoulder joints, called the girdle joints. In some such cases it may be difficult to distinguish the disease from some other rheumatic diseases when there is no back pain present, but the typical back symptoms generally do develop later. Some patients, especially females, may present with neck or upper back pain and stiffness, tenderness of the anterior (front) chest wall, or chest pain that is accentuated on coughing or on taking a deep breath due to inflammation of the joints that attach the ribs to the spine and anterior chest wall. Others may present with inflammation of other structures, such as the eyes, the gut, and the skin, and so their first medical visit may be an eye doctor (ophthalmologist) for an episode of painful acute inflammation of the eye (acute anterior uveitis or AAU for short), discussed in Chapter 6, a gastroenterologist (for symptoms of inflammatory bowel disease (IBD)), or a skin specialist (dermatologist) for psoriasis, as discussed in detail in Chapter 10.

Current terminology

I have explained in the *Preface* that AS belongs to a group of diseases under the term spondyloarthritis (or *SpA* for short). Since AS is predominantly a disease of the axial skeleton, it falls under the newly proposed term *axial* SpA (abbreviated as *axSpA*). A term—radiographic axSpA (r-axSpA)—has sometimes been equated with AS due to the required presence of definite bony structural damage of the SI joints as detected on radiographic (X-ray) examination. But in this book I have used the term AS instead of r-axSpA because it is the most widely used name for this condition.

SpA patients showing involvement predominantly of their "peripheral" limb joints (other than hip and shoulder joints) are labeled as having *predominantly* peripheral SpA, and its best example is psoriatic arthritis (PsA). These two subtypes of axial and peripheral SpA, however, do show some overlapping clinical features (see Figure 2.1), and they also share some of the underlying genetic predisposing factors. Moreover, as discussed in Chapter 10, patients suffering from AAU, IBD, or reactive arthritis have increased risk of developing SpA, either the axial or the peripheral form or both.

Prevalence

AS is present worldwide but with variable prevalence and incidence that are strongly dependent and are directly correlated to the prevalence of HLA-B27 in the general population, as detailed in Chapter 4. For example, it affects approximately up to 1 in 200 (0.5% prevalence) adults of European ancestry, and among northern Arctic communities and Chinese with a wide variation from 0.2 to 0.5%. It is very uncommon in sub-Saharan African populations. I may add that the prevalence figure for the whole group of SpA is even higher as it includes PsA, and SpA associated with IBD and reactive arthritis.

What is its cause?

The cause of AS/axSpA is not yet fully known but carries strong genetic predisposition. Most patients possess a normal gene called *HLA-B27*, that is also present in a very small percent of the general population. (Please note that the term HLA-B27 is italicized only when referring to its gene, but not when it refers to the protein molecule produced by the gene). The genetic predisposition cannot be pinned down to this one gene because many additional genetic factors or genes are also involved (discussed in Chapter 3).

The role of gut microbiome

There are trillions of microorganisms (microbes) comprising viruses, bacteria, and fungi that are present at our "barrier surfaces" (e.g. our gut lining and the skin) that form what we call the human "gut microbiome" and "skin microbiome," respectively. They have evolved to live with us in harmony. The gut microbiome helps digest and convert our food into energy that they also require to survive, and make some key vitamins, such as vitamin K. They also develop and support our immune system to form a frontline of defense to protect us against the harmful microbes. Their effect seems to extend beyond the gut and affect many body functions, even general mood and sleep via the vagus nerve that provides communication between the gut and the brain (the so-called gut–brain axis).

There is a disruption and decreased biodiversity of the gut microbiome in patients with AS, and approximately 60% of the patients have asymptomatic mild gut inflammation, especially among those who also have peripheral joint involvement. Evidence is emerging that the *HLA-B27* gene may have some influence on gut microbiome even in unaffected people. But the presence of asymptomatic gut inflammation in AS patients does not show any clear association with HLA-B27. This supports the existence of some common link between gut inflammation and AS, even independent of HLA-B27.

There are an increasing number of other diseases in which disruptions of the gut microbiome is implicated, ranging from IBD, RA, obesity, diabetes, and colon cancer, while disruption of the skin microbiome may be involved in psoriasis and PsA. It is also important to know that medications, such as anti-biotics, can alter the gut microbiome, and conversely the gut microbiome can metabolize some of the antibiotics and other drugs we take.

Immune system and its role

We possess two main immune strategies against microbial infections: *innate immunity* and *adaptive immunity*. The innate (also called non-specific) immune response is broad and does not need to learn what is dangerous and mostly includes *macrophages*, *neutrophils*, and *dendritic cells* that are equipped with a kind of sensor called pattern recognition receptors (PPRs) that help them quickly trigger defensive strategies by detecting pathogen-associated molecular patterns (PAMPs) that represent overlapping similarities (resemblances) across many disease-causing (pathogenic) microbes. The innate immune response in many cases clears the infection before the adaptive immune response is ready to help out.

The adaptive immune system is more specific because it will recognize exactly the kind of infecting microbe in order to use the exact defensive mechanism needed to get rid of it. This is carried out mainly by *lymphocytes*, and they are split up into *B cells* that produce antibodies and *T cells* that help in getting rid of virus-infected cells. But it takes 10 to 15 days for the T and B cells to acquire that capability and expand in numbers.

The immune cells belonging to both the innate and the adaptive response also build up their memory against the infection so that next time around they more quickly mount a specific (tailor-made) immune response. This adaptive response, that was previously wrongly thought to happen only as part of the adaptive immune system, is called *trained immunity* by which the innate immune cells also improve their ability to deal with the infection the second time around.

Our intestines have more than 350 square feet of inner lining (mucosal membrane or *lamina propria*) that is a major site of development of adaptive immunity. A subset of cells in the gut lining or in the adjacent (mesenteric) regional draining lymph nodes perform a function like that of the thymus gland (located behind the breastbone but in front of the heart that shrinks at the approach of puberty). The mesenteric lymph nodes delete T lymphocytes that can potentially attack body's own organs by a process called "suicidal death" or *apoptosis*. Failure to delete such cells from the gut wall can potentially lead to autoimmune diseases where the body damages itself instead of the harmful invading microbes. Thus, such autoimmunity can also result in sub-clinical (asymptomatic) gut inflammation or even florid IBD.

Any specific environmental trigger for AS remain unknown. Therefore, it has also been proposed that some foreign (non-self-derived) small protein molecules (peptides) may trigger the self-peptide-activated T cells during early life, and this may lead the autoimmune and inflammatory process in later years that results in a disease, including AS.

Laboratory-raised rats genetically engineered to carry the human *HLA-B27* gene have advanced our understanding of how it may predispose humans to AS and related SpA. These so called "HLA-B27 transgenic" rats have been developed in research laboratories that spontaneously develop an inflammatory arthritis that shares many features with the human disease, including sacroiliitis. This illness occurs if they develop diarrhea after they are removed from germ-free (sterile) environment and kept in their natural normal environment. Interestingly, some of these rats without diarrhea develop psoriasis-like skin and nail lesions.

Studies of a mouse model for AS have demonstrated that mechanical strain may trigger inflammation at sites of attachments of ligaments and tendons to bone, known as *entheses* (singular is *enthesis*), and lead to new bone formation that occurs in AS. This is a self-directed inflammation whereby local factors at sites predisposed to disease initiate activation of innate immune cells, including macrophages and neutrophils, that can promote reactive bone remodeling and new bone formation. Thus, biomechanical stress and possible microdamage at entheses and resultant autoinflammatory response independent of adaptive immune system has also been proposed to have a role in development of AS.

Men versus women

AS is diagnosed 2 to 3 times more commonly in men than in women, but there is a preponderance of women among patients with non-radiographic form of axSpA (nr-axSpA), as discussed in the next chapter. Women have a lower intensity of inflammation, but they do not differ from men with regard to physical functional impairment and overall health status. This subject and the prevalence of the disease in women are discussed in Chapter 5.

There is no difference in the age of onset, but the diagnosis in women is delayed significantly longer than among men. For example, a recent review that included 23,883 patients (32.3% were women) from 42 publications reported 8.8 years (range 7.4–10.1) of delay in diagnosis for women versus 6.5 years (range 5.6–7.4) for men. Other factors consistently reported to be associated with longer delays are the patients' lower education levels, younger age at symptom onset and absence of extra-articular (or extra-musculoskeletal) manifestations. Presence of extra-articular manifestation (e.g. recurrent episodes of acute anterior uveitis, presence of psoriasis or IBD), HLA-B27, or a family history of SpA increases the chance of early diagnosis. It is of interest that studies from high-income countries (as defined by the World Bank) have reported longer delays than those from middle-income countries. It is also worth mentioning that in contrast to AS/axSpA, diagnostic delay in PsA was reported to be only 2.6 years.

In an online survey of 2,846 European patients with SpA, women reported higher number of visits to the primary care physicians, physiotherapists, and osteopaths. Neck and upper-back pain, anterior chest wall pain and tenderness (costochondritis), or limb joint involvement may be the main presenting manifestations among women. They also tend to have more anxiety, depression, peripheral joint symptoms and widespread pain. The presence of such clinical features may lead to a misdiagnosis of fibromyalgia (fibrositis) in women suffering from AS/axSpA. There is also a slower and relatively incomplete progression of spinal fusion (ankylosis) among women. This may mean that it takes longer for regression of their pain that often follows complete spinal bony fusion. There are also differences in levels of proinflammatory cytokines and immunological responses. Both men and women respond to treatment with biologics, but women achieve less than a desired level of response and also show a higher discontinuation rate as compared to men.

Hormonal status and fertility are normal in both sexes. Pregnancy usually does not alleviate or change symptoms of AS or it may only cause a temporary aggravation. Childbirth is normal in the absence of severe hip disease. The growth and development of infants and young children are comparable to those of other mothers unaffected with AS. As discussed in a later chapter on management, certolizumab pegol (Cimzia®) is one of the tumor necrosis factor (TNF) inhibitors that can be continued during pregnancy as it does not cross the placenta and therefore the fetus is not exposed to this drug.

Delay in diagnosis

There is an unacceptable delay in the diagnosis of AS/axSpA, partly due to lack of adequate knowledge of many health care providers about its variable clinical presentation, and absence of any validated *diagnostic criteria*. Need for an early diagnosis, including that of nr-axSpA has now become more important because of the availability of increasingly more effective therapies, especially if they are started at early stage of the disease. An early diagnosis also helps avoid unnecessary investigative procedures and inappropriate treatments.

Pointers to early diagnosis are discussed in Chapter 5, and utility of physical examination and appropriate laboratory tests are discussed in Chapter 8. Figure 8.5 shows an algorithm comprising sequential steps that helps experienced clinicians make an early diagnosis of AS/axSpA with increasing levels of confidence from approximately 5% starting at the top of the pyramid to 95% at the base of the pyramid, based on additional features exhibited by the patient. This algorithm does require exclusion of other disease mimicker (look-alike diseases).

New strategies are also being proposed that will assist primary care physicians (PCP) or general practitioners (GP) in early referral of such patients to rheumatologists. Artificial intelligence (AI) methods are being used to recognize disease associated clinical features from very large data sets that may support early identification of patients with suspected diagnosis of AS/axSpA. Algorithm will also be developed in future to facilitate automatic patient referral for those suspected to have early AS/axSpA.

Management

There is no cure yet for AS, but the patients generally respond well to appropriate treatment detailed in Chapters 13 to 20. The newer drug-treatment options include the use of:

◆ Biologic DMARDs (b-DMARDs) that target inflammatory proteins (cytokines), such as TNF and interleukin-17 (IL-17). They are given by injection under the skin or by intravenous infusion.

◆ Targeted synthetic DMARDs (ts-DMARDs) include JAK inhibitors, taken orally as tablets, for the treatment of patients with active AS/axSpA who are intolerant or have had an inadequate response to biologics.

Living with the disease and its socio-economic impact

The disease course is highly variable, and the spine does not always fuse completely when the inflammation stays limited to the SI joints and the lower lumbar spine. Most of the patients can cope well and continue to have a very productive and active lifestyle, especially with an increasingly earlier diagnosis and the use of the above mentioned increasingly more effective (although costly) medications, along with a life-long program of regular physical exercises.

However, some patients may need to modify their lifestyle or their work environment because of worsening impairment of the spinal mobility or worsening hip joint involvement. For example, a manual worker doing heavy lifting and frequent or prolonged bending at work would need a change of job. Most of the socio-economic factors associated with high cost of care are related to uncontrolled disease activity and worsening functional disability. These aspects and effect on life span are discussed in Chapters 21 and 25.

2

Axial spondyloarthritis

 Key points

- Spondyloarthritis (SpA for short) is a name given to a family of chronic inflammatory joint diseases, commonly of young age of onset, that share many clinical features involving the spine and the limbs and are frequently associated with inflammation of other structures, such as the eyes, the gut, and the skin.

- The patients with SpA whose arthritis primarily affects the spine are sub-classified as having "axial SpA" (axSpA), best represented by AS, and those with predominantly limb joints involvement are labeled as having "peripheral SpA," best exemplified by psoriatic arthritis (PsA).

- The term axSpA encompasses both AS (that can be thought of as "radiographic axSpA") and non-radiographic axSpA (nr-axSpA).

- The diagnosis of axSpA relies on the pattern of its clinical manifestations, appropriate laboratory tests, and musculoskeletal imaging.

- Its recognition at an early stage is crucial because of increasingly effective treatment choices that markedly reduce the risk of irreversible structural damage.

- Patients and their caregivers need appropriate counseling and education about the disease to facilitate compliance with the recommended treatment regimens that also includes life-long physical exercises and potential lifestyle modifications to achieve long-term sustained health benefits.

Introduction

I have discussed in the Preface of this book and in **Chapter 1** that spondyloarthritis (abbreviated as SpA) is the name given to a chronic form of inflammatory arthritis of young age of onset that involves the spine and the

Ankylosing Spondylitis and Axial Spondyloarthritis, Second Edition. Muhammad Asim Khan, Oxford University Press.
© Oxford University Press 2023. DOI: 10.1093/oso/9780198864158.003.0002

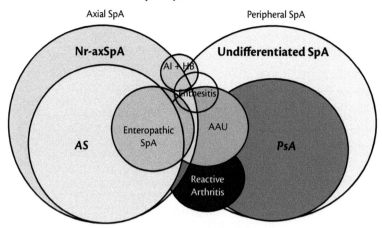

SpA = Spondyloarthritis, Nr-axSpA = non-radiographic axial SpA, PsA = psoriatic arthritis, AAU = acute anterio uveitis, AI+HB = aortic incompetence plus heart block.

Figure 2.1 The two forms of SpA, axial and peripheral.

Adapted from Ozgocmen S and Khan MA. "Current concept of spondyloarthritis: Special emphasis on early referral and diagnosis" *Curr Rheumatol Report.* 2012 Oct;14(5):409–14. © Muhammed Asim Khan

limbs. It can be associated with inflammation of other (non-musculoskeletal) structures, such as the eyes, the gut, and the skin. The patients whose arthritis primarily affects *the axial skeleton* are sub-classified as having "axial SpA" (axSpA for short), best represented by AS that has been discussed in Chapter 1. Whereas those with a predominantly peripheral arthritis (less often the spine) are labeled as having "peripheral SpA," and its best example is psoriatic arthritis (PsA). As shown in Figure 2.1, the two circles (not drawn to scale) representing the two forms of SpA, axial and peripheral, overlap each other, and between them there are smaller circles representing other entities that are discussed in Chapter 10. The prevalence of axSpA has not been well-studied as yet, but a report from France estimated a 0.4% prevalence in their adult population.

Axial SpA

Figure 2.2 schematically represents a unifying concept of axSpA. The decreasing sizes of the three chevrons from the left to the right are meant to

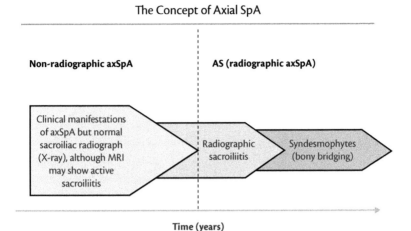

Figure 2.2 This figure schematically shows a unifying concept of a wide clinical spectrum of axSpA. Inflammatory back pain is the leading initial symptom that may be present throughout the disease course without any occurrence of structural damage. The decreasing sizes of the three chevrons from the left to the right are meant to emphasize that only a portion of patients with nr-axSpA will progress to AS (r-axSpA/AS), whereas others may remain as nr-axSpA, perhaps forever or have a self-limiting disease course. This figure also shows that not all patients with AS progress to form syndesmophytes with resulting spinal ankylosis.

Reproduced with permission from Khan MA and van der Linden S. "Axial spondyloarthritis: A better name for an old disease. A step toward uniform reporting." *ACR Open Rheumatology* (ACROR). 2019; and Rudwaleit M, Khan MA, and Sieper J. "The challenge of diagnosis and classification in early ankylosing spondylitis: Do we need new criteria?" *Arthritis & Rheumatism.* 2005;52:1000–8.

emphasize that only a portion of patients with nr-axSpA will progress to AS (r-axSpA). Some may continue to suffer from nr-axSpA throughout the disease course without any occurrence of structural damage or may even have a self-limiting course. Moreover, not all patients with structural damage of their SI joints (sacroiliitis) progress to involve their spine and result in spinal fusion (ankylosis). Although the term "radiographic axSpA" (r-axSpA) is now increasingly being equated with AS, I have preferred to use the term AS that is the widely accepted name for this disease entity.

Non-radiographic axSpA

The term nr-axSpA is often not well understood by the patients nor even by some healthcare providers. This word "non-radiographic" implies that damage in the SI joints and the spine is not visible on X-rays. It needs to be mentioned that the term "radiographic" means X-ray imaging. Magnetic resonance imaging (MRI) involves no use of X-rays, but it can show evidence of inflammation even before any changes can be detected on X-ray examination. This indicates that MRI is more sensitive in detecting presence of inflammation.

Patients with nr-axSpA are characterized by a lower proportion of male patients compared to patients with AS. They also have a lower intensity of inflammation but have similar overall health status. Symptoms usually start in the third decade of life. Some of these patients may only have a series of episodes of aches and pains, coming and going for months, and then become free of all symptoms without any residual damage. But others can progress rapidly, and it is difficult to predict such a progression in an individual patient.

In general, males, smokers, obese individuals, and those with raised level of markers of inflammation (elevated level of C-reactive protein [CRP] and/or erythrocytes sedimentation rate [ESR]), or a high degree of inflammation of their SI joint as detected on MRI, are more likely to progress from nr-axSpA to AS. The most recent report from Germany indicates that 16% of their nr-axSpA patients progress to AS (r-axSpA) within 5 years. The mean time to disease progression was 2.4 years, and predictors included the possession of HLA-B27 along with sacroiliitis on MRI, and male gender.

The clinical recognition (diagnosis) of nr-axSpA is improving, partly due to a better definition of this disease entity and the increasing availability and use of MRI. But MRI is not a very specific indicator of inflammation because similar changes in the SI joints can be seen in many normal individuals and athletes aged less than 45 years, and for up to 6 months in healthy women after childbirth. Therefore, these MRI findings alone can be of limited value in recognizing nr-axSpA unless accompanied by at least some of the other clinical features, the so-called red flags that are discussed later in this chapter.

In patients with late stages of the progressive form of AS/axSpA, the pain in the joints of the back regresses as inflammation is replaced by a healing process that involves new bone formation and ankylosis. This is sometimes referred to as "burning out" of the disease. However, occasional features of AS, such as episodes of eye inflammation (acute anterior uveitis) and heel pain, may continue to occur, suggesting that the disease may not have gone into complete remission. Other patients may continue to suffer from their concomitant psoriasis or IBD.

Early diagnosis is crucial

Early symptoms and pointers to early diagnosis are detailed in Chapter 5. It is very important to recognize the disease at its early stage not only to prevent wrong treatment but also to help set up proper medical management that can minimize symptoms and help reduce functional impairment and risk of disability and deformity. In the absence of any diagnostic criteria or precise disease markers, the diagnosis is based on clinical features, and exclusion of disease "look-alikes." Pointers to early diagnosis are discussed in Chapter 5, and utility of physical examination and appropriate laboratory tests are discussed in Chapter 8.

Classification criteria

If the patients carrying the diagnosis of axSpA wish to take part in research studies, only those who meet the ASAS classification criteria for axSpA will be selected. This criteria set was developed by the ASAS (ASsessment in Axial SpA), a research group of healthcare professionals dedicated to research and education in the field of SpA (<http://www.asas-group.org>). Box 2.1 lists the mnemonic, **SPINEACHE**, we have developed to help recall the clinical features (components) of the ASAS classification criteria. The utility of these criteria

---

Box 2.1 SPINEACHE: A mnemonic for the clinical parameters (components) of the ASAS classification for axial SpA

AxSpA is *classified* by the presence of sacroiliitis on imaging (by radiograph or MRI) **plus** ≥ 1 the clinical parameters listed below. In case there is absence of sacroiliitis, then the presence of HLA-B27 **plus** ≥ 2 other clinical measures are needed.

Mnemonic for the clinical parameters:

SPINEACHE

Sausage digit (dactylitis)

Psoriasis-Positive family history of SpA

Inflammatory back pain

NSAID good response

Enthesitis (heel)

Arthritis

Crohn's/colitis disease—CRP elevated

HLA-B27

Eye (uveitis)

Reproduced with permission from Ozgocmen S, Akgul O, Khan MA. "Mnemonic for assessment of the spondyloarthritis international society criteria" *J Rheumatol.* 2010 Sep;37(9):1978.

---

are currently being validated in an ongoing study called CLassification of Axial SpondyloarthritiS Inception Cohort (CLASSIC) study. *It is important to emphasize that the ASAS criteria are not designed to be used for diagnosis in an individual patient.*

Management

The management of nr-axSpA is very similar to that of AS (discussed in detail in Chapters 13 to 20) and deserves the same level of urgency. It is important to mention here that the approval of certolizumab pegol (Cimzia® is its brand name), a TNF inhibitor, by the European Medicine Agency (EMA) and the US Food and Drug Administration (FDA) to treat nr-axSpA patients is a very good news for women of child-bearing age suffering from nr-axSpA (and AS or other forms of SpA) because this treatment can be continued during pregnancy and the subsequent breast-feeding period as the drug does not cross the placenta (and therefore the fetus is not exposed to the drug) or enter the mother's milk.

3

What is the underlying cause? *HLA-B27* and other disease-predisposing genes

 Key points

♦ AS/axSpA has a strong genetic predisposition, best exemplified by its association with a perfectly normal gene called *HLA-B27*, carried by a small percentage of the general population. But only a tiny minority (<5%) of the HLA-B27-positive people get AS or related forms of SpA.

♦ Presence of HLA-B27 is not a prerequisite because people lacking it can also suffer from these diseases. Testing for HLA-B27 can be helpful when there is diagnostic uncertainty after thorough clinical evaluation.

♦ *HLA-B27* provides approximately 20% of the total genetic risk and there are ~140 additional such genes or genetic variants; they all interact with each other and possibly with non-genetic (environmental) factors to result in disease.

♦ There is a disruption of the gut microbiome and up to 60% of the patients with AS have asymptomatic inflammation in the gut. This supports the existence of a link between gut inflammation and AS.

♦ An increasingly better understanding of the cause of AS and related forms of SpA has already led to an increasing number of new and very effective therapies.

Ankylosing Spondylitis and Axial Spondyloarthritis, Second Edition. Muhammad Asim Khan, Oxford University Press.
© Oxford University Press 2023. DOI: 10.1093/oso/9780198864158.003.0003

Introduction

We do not yet know the precise cause of AS or what triggers it. This disease is not contagious or infectious and is not due to injury or athletic activity. The underlying cause is multi-factorial, i.e., there are multiple predisposing factors, including genetic and non-genetic (environmental) factors, that influence the timing of the onset as well as the clinical manifestations of the disease.

Presence of genetic predisposition had long been suspected because of occasional occurrence of the disease in multiple members of the same family. The discovery of a remarkable association of a normal gene named *HLA-B27* with AS and related forms of SpA was first reported in 1973. It helped to revitalize the clinical and genetic studies of these disorders and broadened our understanding of their wider clinical spectrum. However, we still do not know exactly how *HLA-B27* gene plays its role in disease predisposition. It contributes approximately 20% of the total genetic risk and there is substantial evidence that it has a direct role in enhancing genetic susceptibility to AS, along with ~140 additional genetic factors that influence disease susceptibility, expression, and/or severity. Current research is focusing on identification of additional genes and also epigenetic (environmental) factors (that, unlike genes, are reversible and can often be modulated) or infections that may trigger the disease.

It is important to emphasize that possession of the *HLA-B27* gene is not always required for AS or related SpA to occur as people lacking this gene can also get these diseases. Moreover, although people born with the *HLA-B27* gene in the general population are more predisposed, only a tiny minority (<5%) of them get AS or related forms of SpA. But this percentage is higher among children who inherit *HLA-B27* gene from a parent with AS.

What is HLA-B27?

HLA stands for human leucocyte antigens. These are cell surface proteins that vary from person to person and are the products of genes located on chromosome number 6. The locations (or loci) of these genes are given the letters A, B, C, D, and so on. There are thousands of varieties of the HLA genes at some of these loci in the general population and it is very difficult to find two genetically unrelated but HLA-identical individuals (i.e., possessing an exactly identical combination of these variations).

These genes and their products, i.e., the HLA molecules, are grouped into two broad classes called HLA class I and class II. HLA-B27 is so named because its gene is located at the B locus belonging to the HLA class I group and is assigned the number 27. The name is italicized (*HLA-B27*) when it refers to the gene rather than its product expressed on the surface as a protein molecule (HLA-B27).

When a cell gets infected by a microorganism it will display on its surface the foreign peptides (a few amino acids linked together) derived from it in combination with HLA class I molecules, such as HLA-B27, in the same way as it handles normal self-derived peptides. For example, viral peptides presented by HLA molecule activate certain T cells that have "receptors" on their surface that allow them to "see" at a chemical level this viral peptide and destroy the infected cells. These T cells are called CD8 + cytotoxic T cells that specifically target the foreign infecting microbes (bacteria, fungi, or viruses). Figure 3.1 shows such a peptide, usually 8 to 10 amino acids long, presented in the pocket of HLA-B27 molecule for

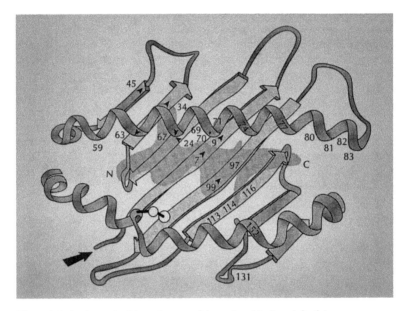

Figure 3.1 A schematic ribbon diagram of the antigen binding cleft of the most prevalent natural variant (subtype) of HLA-B27 molecule. A nine amino-acid long peptide is bound in the cleft, anchored at sites marked by black arrow heads, and the letters N (amino) and C (carboxy) indicate its two ends. The bound peptide is presented by HLA-B27 to CD8 positive T cells. The numbers indicate the locations of the amino acid differences (substitutions) among the first 12 subtypes of HLA-B27 that were known in the early 1990s.

Reproduced with permission from Khan MA. "Spondyloarthropathies" *Curr Opin Rheumatol.* 1994;6:351–3.

Prevalence of HLA-B27 in world populations

recognition by CD8 + cytotoxic T cells specific for that peptide. The general public has become more familiar with these cells on reading about the virus causing the COVID-19 pandemic.

Prevalence of HLA-B27 in world populations

The prevalence of HLA-B27 in the general population varies markedly among the different native ethnic/racial groups throughout the world (Figure 3.2). Its prevalence is much higher among native or "First Nation" North American tribes and circumpolar native population in Eurasia. For simplicity, the percentage prevalence numbers in this figure are rounded off. Not shown is the effect of European colonization, accompanied by migration (settlement) and associated decimation of the native inhabitants that has resulted in the 6% overall prevalence of HLA-B27 in the current population in North America, 5% in South America, and 7% in Australia. In the US, on average, approximately 7% of "non-Hispanic whites", 5% of Hispanics and 2% of "blacks" (African Americans) possess the *HLA-B27* gene.

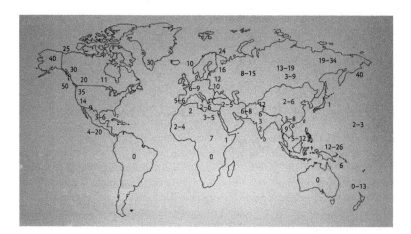

Figure 3.2 The prevalence (%) of HLA-B27 in native (indigenous) genetically unmixed populations of the world. Not shown in this Figure is the effect of colonization and migration by the Europeans so that the general prevalence of HLA-B27 is approximately 6% in the current populations in North America, 5% in South America, and 7% in Australia.

Reproduced with permission from Khan MA. "Editorial overview: Spondyloarthropathies" *Curr Opin Rheumatol.* 1998;10:279–81.

As shown in Table 4.1 and in Table 4.2, AS and related forms of SpA are more common in populations with a relatively higher prevalence of HLA-B27, such as the circumpolar native populations, including Inuits in the US and Canada. The converse is also true because the *HLA-B27* gene and AS are both absent among the surviving Australian indigenous (formerly called "aboriginal") populations of unmixed genetic ancestry. The native inhabitants of unmixed genetic ancestry in South America and southern part of the African continent also virtually lack this gene and AS, But there are some exceptions to this generalization, e.g., certain West African population groups have 2–4% prevalence of HLA-B27 but occurrence of AS is quite uncommon.

Inheritance of genes

Our cells contain a set of 22 pairs of chromosomes (named autosomes) and one pair of sex chromosomes assigned the letters X and Y; 23 of these 46 chromosomes we inherit from our father and the other 23 from our mother. Each chromosome is a tiny but a very long tightly rolled thread-like structure that contains a set of our genes. The father contributes his set of 22 autosomes and his X or a Y sex chromosome to the offspring, while the mother contributes her set of 22 autosomes and one of her two X chromosome. Each son has an X and a Y sex chromosome, and each daughter has two X chromosomes. Male genes on the Y chromosomes allow male cells to function in a different way from female cells. Thus, it is not surprising that disease occurrences and their clinical manifestations can differ in the two sexes.

Inheritance of *HLA-B27* gene

As mentioned earlier, the HLA genes are present on chromosome 6. Thus, as a result, each of us has an HLA-B location on each of our two chromosomes 6. Someone is said to be HLA-B27-positive if the gene for it is present at HLA-B location on either one or both of these chromosomes. If a parent has HLA-B27 at one of these two HLA-B gene locations, then there is a 1 in 2 chance that the offspring will inherit this gene. In a much less likely possibility of both parents possessing an *HLA-B27* gene, there will then be 1 in 4 chance that their offspring will inherit this gene from both parents (such a child will be HLA-B27 homozygous), 1 in 2 chance of inheriting the gene from only one parent (HLA-B27 heterozygous), and 1 in 4 chance of not inheriting the gene (HLA-B27-negative).

HLA-B27 testing in disease diagnosis

AS/axSpA and related SpA can often be readily diagnosed based on clinical history, physical examination, and use of X-ray imaging or MRI. Therefore HLA-B27 test is not needed for diagnosis in every patient, and these diseases also occur in people who lack this gene. Moreover, a negative test result for HLA-B27 does not completely exclude the presence of the disease. Conversely, because the *HLA-B27* gene is present in a significant percentage of the healthy general population, a positive test result does not mean that someone has the disease. So, typing for HLA-B27 should not be considered a routine, diagnostic, confirmatory, or screening test for AS in patients with back pain in the general population.

A knowledge of the presence of HLA-B27 can sometimes be valuable as an aid to diagnosis but only when performed in the context of the clinical setting and *a priori* (pre-test) likelihood of the disease. It also needs to be emphasized that the prevalence of HLA-B27 and the strength of its disease association varies markedly with the different forms of SpA, and also among the many ethnic and racial groups worldwide. For example, more than 90% of Scandinavian patients with AS are HLA-B27-positive, but this percentage drops to 75% among patients from countries surrounding the Mediterranean Sea and as low as 50% among African American patients.

Clinicians who understand the principles of probability reasoning order the HLA-B27 test only in a toss-up clinical situation, e.g., for a patient with suggestive clinical picture and an elevated ESR or CRP in the presence of normal or equivocal SI joint X-rays. The positive test result for HLA-B27 in this clinical situation would further increase the likelihood of nr-axSpA. On the other hand, a negative HLA-B27 test result alone would not rule out the disease and may require further diagnostic clarity by ordering MRI to look for inflammation of the SI joints.

Genetic counseling

It is important for the doctor to obtain the patient's family history as it is not unusual for more than one person in a family to be affected with AS or a related form of SpA because of the strong genetic predisposition. As discussed earlier, if a parent possesses HLA-B27, ~50% of the children will inherit HLA-B27.

A patient of northern European heritage suffering from AS without any associated psoriasis or IBD (who has >85% chance of possessing the HLA-B27 gene) may ask, "What is the risk of my children developing AS and can anything be done to prevent this?" We have very recently published the results of our long-term family study lasting 35 years. The results indicate that the HLA-B27-positive children of an HLA-B27-positive parent with AS carry a substantial (~25%) risk of developing axSpA (AS or nr-axSpA) during their lifetime, and it is even a little higher among HLA-B27-positive children of an HLA-B27-positive affected mother. However, it is important to emphasize that ~75% of HLA-B27-positive and virtually all of the HLA-B27-negative children will remain free from this disease if there is no occurrence of psoriasis or IBD in the family. We do not know how to completely prevent this disease from occurring. However, an early diagnosis is essential for a good outcome, given the availability of much more effective, although costly, treatments.

This patient may then ask, "Should I have all my children tested for the HLA-B27?" Generally speaking, the answer is no because most of the 50% children that are expected to inherit this gene from him will remain un-affected during their lifetime. Moreover, one may unwittingly introduce an-other ailment, what I call "HLA-B27-itis," because knowing that the child has HLA-B27, the parents may worry unnecessarily for many years, and the child may get a wrong diagnostic label of juvenile SpA/axSpA for any joint symptoms or sports-related injury. Children who are born with HLA-B27 but remain unaffected may suffer indirectly in the future if the information about their test result enters their medical records and thus becomes avail-able to health insurance agencies or future potential employers, who may misuse such information.

The risk of disease occurrence among the children of HLA-B27-negative pa-tients is very low, unless other diseases, such as IBD or psoriasis, are present in the family. If a son or a daughter of a parent living with AS (possessing or lacking HLA-B27) develops symptoms or signs that the parent, based on his or her personal experience as a patient, suspects to be due to AS/axSpA or related SpA, or the child develops acute anterior uveitis, psoriasis or IBD, prompt rheumatologic consultation can lead to an early diagnosis and initi-ation of effective treatment.

The role of HLA-B27 and other disease-predisposing genes

As discussed earlier, a greater prevalence of AS is observed in HLA-B27-positive first-degree relatives of AS patients than in HLA-B27-positive random controls from the general population. This suggests that AS results from an influence of multiple genes. This is medically termed as a "genetically heterogeneous" disease, i.e., there are additional genetic predisposing factors. Recent genome-wide association studies (GWAS) have identified about 140 genetic variants, including HLA-B27, that together explain >30% genetic risk for AS. HLA-B27 alone contributes approximately 20% of this risk.

Different subtypes of HLA-B27

So far more than 240 different subtypes of HLA-B27 have been reported. An overwhelming majority of them are very rare and were only recognized with the discovery of the modern molecular rather than the old serological typing methods. In the current scientific nomenclature, the use of this modern method is indicated by the insertion of an * between B and 27. The distribution of these different HLA-B*27 subtypes varies among the various world populations. For example, the HLA-B*27:05 subtype is the most common subtype worldwide. However, the Han Chinese have a higher prevalence of HLA-B*27:04 than HLA-B*27:05. AS has been observed to occur in individuals born with any of the more common HLA-B27 subtypes studied thus far, except that two subtypes seem to be, at the most, only very weakly associated with AS. They are HLA-B*27:06, found in south-east Asian populations, and HLA-B*27:09, a rare subtype observed primarily among Italian populations, especially those living on the island of Sardinia.

The role of non-genetic factors

The more you inherit the various disease-predisposing genes the more likely you are to suffer from AS/axSpA or related forms of SpA. However, it still requires some, yet unknown, environmental (i.e., non-genetic) trigger(s) for the disease to start. Better understanding of how some of the genes interact with non-genetic factors to trigger diseases has already led to some of the new and more effective therapies. Some forms of SpA, particularly reactive arthritis (Reiter's syndrome), discussed later in this book, can be triggered after an episode of infection in the genitourinary tract or the gut by certain bacteria. However, most patients with AS do not evolve after a reactive arthritis like illness. This suggests differences in the environmental triggers for these two forms of SpA.

Thus far we do not know any specific bacterial or other microbial trigger for AS, and there was a time when gut infection with *Klebsiella* bacteria was wrongly proposed as a trigger. There is very strong evidence for a disruption in the composition of microbiome (the microorganisms that normally start living peacefully on and in our bodies the moment we are born and for the rest of our lives) can trigger inflammatory arthritis, including AS and related forms of SpA, especially in genetically susceptible individuals. This was discussed in Chapter 1.

What have we learnt from all this research?

An individual born with HLA-B27 destined to develop AS may be predisposed to disruption of his/her gut microbiome for some reasons; and this activates their immune response to trigger the disease if they are genetically susceptible (prone) for it. Perhaps, a microorganism-derived peptide or an HLA-B27-derived protein itself gets bound to HLA-B27, and thus provides a trigger for the disease to happen. But it needs to be restated that the disease does occur also in individuals lacking HLA-B27.

People who have inherited certain HLA types are better at defending against certain pathogens but at the same time they may be more vulnerable to certain other infections or diseases. For example, an individual born with HLA-B27 can mount a better response against many viruses, such as the hepatitis C virus, but can be more vulnerable to getting AS/axSpA and related forms of SpA. It may be of interest for readers to know there is another class of HLA molecules called the *HLA class II*, and one of them called HLA-DR4 is strongly associated with RA.

4

Disease prevalence

 Key points

- Disease *prevalence* is defined as the number of disease cases present in a particular population at a given time and can be reported as a percentage (%). Disease *incidence* defines the number of new cases that develop during a specified period of time.

- Prevalence is a more suitable measure to compare burden imposed by a disease and is influenced by both the rate at which new cases are occurring (incidence) and the average duration of the disease (time from diagnosis until the patient recovers, dies, or cannot be traced due to various reasons).

- Large-scale and well-done epidemiological studies to establish the worldwide prevalence and incidence of AS/axSpA are very scant. The results vary widely because they are influenced by ethnicity, race, HLA-B27 prevalence in the population, study design, and the methods used for disease ascertainment.

- Studies of adult populations of European and Chinese descent suggest an up to 0.5% prevalence of AS. Men are 2 to 3 times more likely to suffer from AS, but nr-axSpA is more common in women.

Introduction

Musculoskeletal conditions affect people across all ages around the world. Recognition and understanding of the disease burden on the society is needed for determining the optimal healthcare needs of the population, and to ensure efficient allocation and effective management of available healthcare resources.

Ankylosing Spondylitis and Axial Spondyloarthritis, Second Edition. Muhammad Asim Khan, Oxford University Press.
© Oxford University Press 2023. DOI: 10.1093/oso/9780198864158.003.0004

Disease occurrence is assessed by two types of measures: prevalence and incidence. Disease *prevalence* answers, "How many people have the disease in a particular population at a given time?" During the COVID-19 pandemic, the public has become quite familiar with this term. There is another term called "disease *incidence*" that defines the number of new cases that develop during a specified period of time. Prevalence is a more suitable measure to compare burden imposed by a disease and is influenced by both the rate at which new cases are occurring (incidence) and the average duration of the disease (time from diagnosis until the patient recovers, dies, or cannot be traced due to various reasons). It is also helpful in assessing the underlying cause of the disease and identifying its risk factors.

Prevalence and incidence of AS/axSpA

One of the long, ongoing debates concerns the prevalence and incidence of AS/axSpA. The earliest medical center-based studies gave very conservative estimates since many individuals with AS/axSpA have relatively mild disease and they do not seek medical care. Moreover, now we know that any prevalence and incidence studies of AS can be markedly influenced by multiple factors, such as the differences in the methodologies used, the disease definition, and the prevalence of the *HLA-B27* gene.

There are a few large-scale epidemiological studies, but they have yielded variable results. AxSpA prevalence was estimated at 0.4% of the French adult population. A study in the US reviewed pelvic X-rays of 5,013 adults participating in the 2009–2010 US National Health and Nutritional Examination Survey (NHANES) reported a 0.9% to 1.4% prevalence of axSpA. But these investigators had no information about the HLA-B27 status and the MRI findings of the SI joints of these patients that are required to calculate the prevalence of axSpA according to the latest validated criteria.

Another US study relying on searching the billing codes in a computerized database of a non-profit health delivery system suggested a 0.23% national prevalence of axSpA, but the authors did not have the ability to identify undiagnosed cases. Another US study estimated national prevalence of axSpA to be 0.7%, subdivided into 0.35% for AS and 0.35% also for nr-axSpA. This study was based on a review of the medical records of 861 randomly selected patients (age 18 to 44 years) with chronic back pain being followed at more than 100 rheumatology offices.

AS is very uncommon among Japanese (with less than 1% prevalence of HLA-B27) as compared to Chinese and Koreans (with 4 to 6% prevalence of HLA-B27 in their general population). The HLA-B27 gene in the US population is approximately 3 times less prevalent among African Americans versus "non-Hispanic whites," and correspondingly they less often suffer from AS. Table 4.1 shows selected examples of data showing direct correlation of HLA-B27 and AS/axSpA in the general population. In an old study of Haida native tribal community living on an island in British Columbia, a province of Canada, reported that 6–10% of adults had AS. A subsequent study in this community reported a 50% prevalence of HLA-B27 in the general population (highest in world).

A British study of 971 randomly selected adults who had consulted their primary care physicians for their low back pain were mailed a validated questionnaire for AS/axSpA. The respondents describing inflammatory back pain were then invited for a clinical evaluation, supplemented with HLA-B27 testing and imaging studies. The investigators estimated a 0.3% prevalence for axSpA in the general adult population; this includes a 0.15% prevalence for AS. In a smaller study from Turkey that was based on a survey of 381 university employees; and those with inflammatory back pain underwent a full clinical

Table 4.1 Selected examples of data prior to the year 1998 showing direct correlation of HLA-B27 and AS/axSpA in the general population

Populations	HLA-B27 (%)	Prevalence of AS (%)		Prevalence of SpA including AS (%)	
		General Population	B27(+) Population	General Population	B27(+) Population
Circumpolar native populations in Eurasia, Inuits in Canada and US, and Chukchis in Siberia)	24–40	0.4 – 1.8	1.6–6.8	2–3.4	4.2*
Haida natives (Canada)	50	6–10	20		
Northern Norwegians	14	1.1	6.7		

*All these patients had radiographically diagnosed AS.
Source: data from Khan MA. "A worldwide overview—The epidemiology of HLA-B27 and associated spondyloarthritides" in Calin A and Taurog J (eds), *The Spondylarthritides*. Oxford: Oxford University Press, 1998, 17–26.

Table 4.2 The pooled prevalence rates (%) of AS and SpA in the various regions of the world published prior to 1998

Populations		AS	SpA (including AS)
North America		0.20	1.35
Europe		0.25	0.54
Middle East/ North Africa		0.11	0.32
Asia	South	0.06	0.22
	South-East	0.07	0.20
	China—East	0.16	0.79
Sub-Saharan Africa		0.02	
South America		0.14	

Source: data from Khan MA. "A worldwide overview—The epidemiology of HLA-B27 and associated spondyloarthritides" in Calin A and Taurog J (eds), *The Spondylarthritides*. Oxford: Oxford University Press, 1998, 17–26.

evaluation that included HLA-B27 testing and imaging studies. These investigators estimated a 1.3% prevalence for axSpA (that includes 0.5% prevalence for AS) among Turkish adult population. A relatively recent study from Slovenia reported an estimated annual incidence rate of SpA to be 14.3 per 100,000 adults (16.2 among men and 12.5 among women). Table 4.2 provides the pooled global prevalence rates of AS and SpA (including AS) in the various regions of the world prior to 1998.

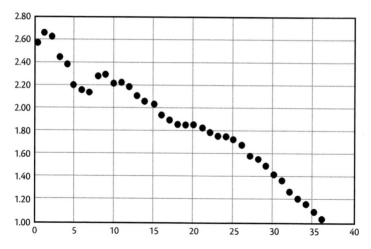

Figure 4.1 The yearly change in the ratio between men and women with AS is shown in the vertical axis, while the horizontal axis shows follow-up observations, listed at 5-year intervals, since 1980. The last observation was at the end of 2016, covering a span of 37 years.

Source: data from Baumberger H and Khan MA. "Gradual progressive change to equal prevalence of ankylosing spondylitis among males and females in Switzerland: Data from the Swiss Ankylosing Spondylitis Society (SVMB)" *Ann Rheum Dis* 2017;76 (Suppl 2) 929. (Presented at the Annual European Congress of Rheumatology EULAR 2017, Madrid, Spain. June 14–17, 2017. DOI:10.1136/annrheumdis-2017-eular.3961.

Occurrence among women

Data from Switzerland indicated that AS/axSpA was 2.6 times more common in men than women in 1980, and this ratio has shown a gradual decline since then, so that by December 2016 the disease was found to be equally prevalent among men and women (Figure 4.1). This has resulted from increasingly more accurate disease definition, improved classification criteria, easy availability of MRI, and better recognition of nr-axSpA that is more common in women. This change is also helped by Switzerland's good healthcare system, and a greater awareness of the disease among the general public, facilitated in part by the efforts of the Swiss Ankylosing Spondylitis Society. It is of interest that a study from the Canadian province of Ontario with a much shorter study duration reported that in 1995 the disease was 1.7 times more common among men than women, and that ratio decreased significantly to 1.4 in the year 2000, 1.3 in 2005, and finally 1.21 by the year 2010.

5

Early symptoms and pointers to early diagnosis

 Key points

◆ Back pain is very prevalent in the general population, and AS is not its commonest cause. An insidious (gradual) onset of back pain and stiffness felt in the lower back and buttock area in a teenager or a young adult is usually the initial symptom of AS/axSpA.

◆ These symptoms are worsened by prolonged inactivity, especially at late hours of the night or on waking up in the morning, and they tend to be eased by physical exercise, hot shower, or after taking non-steroidal anti-inflammatory drugs (NSAIDs).

◆ Some patients may only have relatively mild backache, others have symptoms that may come and go over many months, without troubling them enough to seek medical help. Most people with AS/axSpA first seek medical help when the back pain and stiffness become persistent and troublesome and a major impediment to good sleep.

◆ Others may first seek medical help because of inflammation at some other sites, which then turns out to be associated with AS. For example, the patient may have psoriasis, IBD, or one or more episodes of acute inflammation of the eye (acute iritis).

◆ A few patients may present with pain in the hip (groin) or knee joint, or tenderness of some bones, such as the chest wall or the heels.

◆ Unless the physician has ample clinical experience and a high index of suspicion, many cases will be missed, especially at early stages of the disease when proper medical management can help alleviate not only the symptoms but also help reduce the risk of long-term disability and deformity.

Ankylosing Spondylitis and Axial Spondyloarthritis, Second Edition. Muhammad Asim Khan, Oxford University Press. © Oxford University Press 2023. DOI: 10.1093/oso/9780198864158.003.0005

Introduction

Back pain is very prevalent in the general population, and up to 80% of the general population in the US will have a lower back problem of some type at least once in their lifetime. It is also the most frequent reason for temporary disability for young persons under 45 years of age, and is often called "mechanical back pain" or "non-specific back pain," Most of these people recover within weeks or up to 6 months, regardless of any medical care or intervention. AS/axSpA is not the commonest cause of chronic back pain. However, an insidious (gradual) onset of backpain and stiffness *for no apparent reason* in *late adolescence or early adulthood* among males and females is usually the initial symptom of AS/axSpA (discussed in Chapters 1 and 2). This "inflammatory back pain" results from inflammation of the SI joints (sacroiliitis) and the spine (spondylitis) and is eased on physical exercise or intake of NSAIDs.

Early symptoms

Most people with AS/axSpA complain of dull ache that is felt deep in the buttock area overlying the SI joints and in the lower back. At first it may be intermittent or on one side only, or alternate between sides; however, within a few months it generally becomes persistent (chronic) and is felt on both sides (bilateral). Gradually this lower back pain and stiffness worsens as the inflammation extends up the lumbar spine. The patients first seek medical help when their back pain and stiffness become persistent and troublesome and may be a major impediment to good sleep. General fatigue and tiredness may be a major concern for many patients, but these symptoms are also independently associated with depression, anxiety, obesity, and lack of physical activity. Some patients, more often women, may primarily complain of fleeting muscle aches, tender areas over the front of the chest and upper back and neck that may occasionally be misdiagnosed as "fibromyalgia" or "fibrositis."

The disease may sometimes be associated with inflammation of hip or shoulder joints (called the girdle joints), and less often the more peripheral limb joints, such as knees, ankles, or elbows. In fact, for some people, the first symptoms may not be back pain but painful girdle joints (hip (groin) and shoulder joints) or lower limb joints, especially in the juvenile onset form of the disease. Others may present with bone tenderness, such as in the heels, that may make it difficult to stand or walk for long, especially on a hard or rough surface, or inflammation of the Achilles tendon.

Some patients may present with chest pain and tenderness, or notice worsening of the pain on taking a deep breath. This results from inflammation and gradual fusion of the joint attaching the ribs to the thoracic spine in the back and to the anterior (front) chest wall. Others may visit their doctor after an episode of acute inflammation of the eye (acute anterior uveitis), psoriasis or symptoms of IBD; and their back symptoms may be very mild or absent. However, the typical back symptoms of AS/axSpA do develop later.

Pointers to early diagnosis

The inflammatory back pain of early AS/axSpA (Box 1.1), as mentioned earlier, is usually a dull ache that is difficult to localize, felt deep in the buttock or lower back, and associated with stiffness and muscle spasms. Some patients may have tenderness over lower back and the SI joints. Physical activity or a hot shower helps minimize back pain and stiffness, whereas exposure to cold or dampness may make the symptoms worse. The back symptoms are typically worse at late hours of the night and on waking up in the morning ("morning stiffness") because their long period of inactivity usually exacerbates the pain and stiffness. The patients may find it necessary to get out of bed at night with considerable difficulty and move about for a few minutes or exercise before going back to bed. The resultant inadequate sleep can be associated with general tiredness and fatigue during the day.

Most cases of AS/axSpA can be diagnosed, or at least initially suspected, based on a good medical history and a thorough clinical examination. It is important to emphasize that obtaining the patient's history should take precedence over physical examination because performing the examination without a good clinical history may not provide much help in supporting or refuting the physician's early clinical suspicion. Here is a list of questions that healthcare providers should ask the person presenting with back pain to differentiate the "inflammatory back pain" due to AS and related forms of SpA from the vastly much more common "non-specific" or "mechanical" back pain that results from other causes:

- Where is your pain the worst; in your back or your legs?

- Have you had the same symptoms before, and at what age did they first begin?

- Is your pain constant or intermittent, and is there ever a time when you are completely pain free, even for a short time?

- Does your pain typically get worse at late hours of the night or wake up with back stiffness that lasts more than half an hour?

- Does prolonged rest, physical inactivity, or special positions ease your pain?

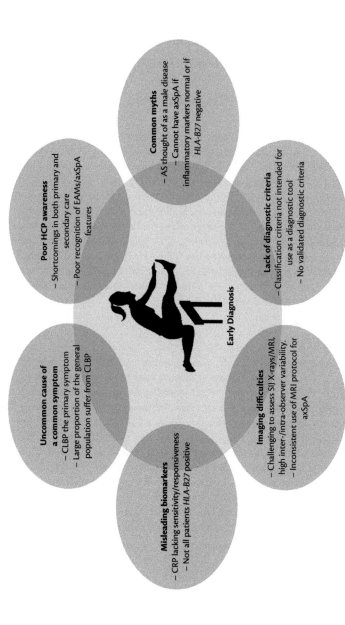

Figure 5.1 Hurdles to the path to early diagnosis.

Adapted with permission from Barnett R, Ingram T, and Sengupta R. "Axial spondyloarthritis 10 years on: Still looking for the lost tribe" *Rheumatology.* 2020 Oct;59(Suppl 4)iv25–iv37.

- Does bending forward typically make your pain worse or cause shooting pain going down your leg?

- How has it affected your day-to-day activities?

- Has there been a change in your bowel or bladder function since your pain started?

- What treatments have you had, and did you notice any benefit from any of them?

During a thorough physical examination, the clinician should look for the presence of objective signs of inflammation affecting the SI joints and the spine, as well as the extremities, skin, and the eyes, in addition to the routine physical check-up. There may be tenderness or pain caused by either direct firm pressure over the SI joints or by physically stressing these joints by some physical maneuvers. The range of chest expansion, and mobility of the spine, including the neck, needs to be measured. The diagnosis of AS also involves musculoskeletal imaging (X-rays, MRI, or low-radiation CT) and laboratory tests to help exclude other possible causes of symptoms. These are described in Chapters 8 and 9. Figure 5.1 nicely summarizes the various hurdles the patients may have to face in the path to early diagnosis. Some of these hurdles are faced more often by female patients (discussed in Chapter 1).

Disease course

The disease course is very variable; some may get transient generalized episodic flares of back pain and stiffness with periods in between when there are mostly asymptomatic ("in remission"). Generally, the chronic inflammatory back pain persists for decades due to active inflammation if not adequately controlled by the treatment they are receiving. In some patients the spine may not fuse completely because their disease may stay limited to the SI joints and extend only to the lower (lumbar) spine. Others develop extension of inflammation to the upper back, chest wall, shoulder girdle, and the neck that results in progressive decrease in range of motion of these sites and progressive diminution of chest expansion. The bony ankylosis of the spine and associated osteoporosis usually progresses over time and results in varying degrees of diminishing spinal mobility and progressive forward stooping (kyphosis) of the whole spine, including the neck.

6

Eye inflammation (acute anterior uveitis)

➲ Key points

♦ Acute inflammation in the front (anterior) eye components is called acute anterior uveitis. One or more such episodes can occur at some time during AS/axSpA, and the recurrent episodes can involve the same or the other eye.

♦ It is the most common site of inflammation occurring outside of the musculoskeletal (bones, joints, and tendons) inflammation caused by AS/axSpA.

♦ Typical symptoms include painful red eye, associated with excessive tearing, and an uncomfortable feeling on looking directly at a bright light.

♦ It is advised that patients should promptly see an ophthalmologist (eye specialist) for diagnosis and prompt treatment.

♦ The patients usually respond very well to local eye drops of corticosteroids and medicines that dilate the pupil (mydriatics). Risk of recurrence is markedly decreased in patients receiving monoclonal TNF inhibitors for their AS/axSpA.

♦ If left untreated or treated inadequately, uveitis may cause some degree of permanent impairment of the eyesight.

The structure (anatomy) of the eye

The eye is a hollow three-layered sphere filled with fluid (vitreous gel). The outer layer is called the sclera (the white of the eye) with a transparent front part called the cornea (the most frontal transparent [clear] part of the eye). The innermost

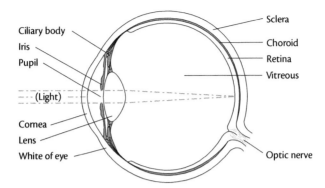

Figure 6.1 Anatomic structure shown as a vertical section in the middle of the eyeball (side view). Not labelled in this figure is the region called macula that has a small central pit called fovea where the light rays get focused on to the retina.

layer is the retina, and the middle layer is the uvea. The front part of uvea is the iris, the colored part of the eye that surrounds the pupil (the dark round area at the center of the eye); and its adjacent structure called the ciliary body (where some of the eye fluid is produced) that is attached to the lens (Figure 6.1). The choroid is the back part of the uvea that brings blood to the retina.

The pupil controls the light waves entering the eye and the lens focusses them on to a small pit called the fovea for crisp vision. This is the most sensitive part of the retina, located in the center of a small area called the macula in the central part of the retina in the back of the eye. These two structures are not labeled in the figure. The optic nerve then carries the sight signals from the eye to the brain.

When any part of uvea becomes inflamed it is called *uveitis*, which means inflamed uvea. *Iritis* is the term used when the inflammation is restricted to the iris, while the term *anterior uveitis* means inflammation of the iris as well as the ciliary body. The term *acute* refers to a short-term illness of abrupt onset and lasting less than 3 months. Acute iritis, an old term, is still sometimes used, but the more precise term is *acute anterior uveitis* (AAU) because the acute inflammation affects both the iris and the ciliary body) or *acute anterior non-granulomatous uveitis* (to indicate the type of inflammation).

Symptoms of acute anterior uveitis

One or more episodes of acute inflammation in the eye is the most common site of inflammation occurring outside of the bones, joints, and tendons that form the main places affected by the disease. The patient initially may feel that something is going wrong with the eye for a day or two before the inflammation worsens. Then the patient notices pain in the eye, associated with redness, excessive tearing, an uncomfortable feeling on looking directly at a bright light, and blurriness of vision resulting from a build-up of inflammatory cells and proteins in the front part of the eye. The pupil looks constricted (small pupil) because of inflammation results in swelling of the iris. Use of dark glasses may decrease sensitivity to bright light.

There can be recurrent episodes of eye inflammation, and each episode typically affects one eye only, but the next episode may affect the same or the other eye ("flip-flop" from one eye to the other). It can occur in both males and females and is most common in people who possess HLA-B27, and mostly occur at 15 to 50 years of age. Besides genetic factors, environmental factors that are as yet undefined also play a role. Use of monoclonal TNF-inhibitors (discussed in Chapter 19) for the patient's AS/axSpA has lessened its occurrence or recurrence. Prior to the advent of this therapy, approximately 25% of patients used to have one or more episode of AAU within the first 10 years of AS. This percentage gradually used to exceed 40% in HLA-B27-positive patients after 40 years of suffering from AS. AAU may occur before the onset of AS/axSpA or even when the disease is minimally active or in remission, and the likelihood is markedly reduced among patients already on monoclonal TNF-inhibitor therapy.

Treatment of uveitis

It is strongly advised that the patient should promptly (within a day or two) see an ophthalmologist (eye specialist) for diagnosis and treatment, especially if the eye pain is associated with blurred vision and redness. The inflammation and associated symptoms usually resolve within 2 to 4 weeks with appropriate treatment that includes use of eye drops to dilate the pupil, to keep the inflamed iris away from the lens and the cornea and decrease pain (by reducing muscle spasm in the ciliary body), and corticosteroid eyedrops to control the inflammation. These corticosteroid eyedrops are initially used very frequently, even hourly, depending on the severity of the inflammation. As stated earlier, the likelihood of getting an attack of uveitis is markedly reduced among patients already on monoclonal TNF-inhibitor therapy.

A few patients may require treatment with a brief course of corticosteroid tablets or TNF-inhibitors or other immune-suppressant drugs for their severe or more widespread uveitis that may have failed to show adequate response. The inflammatory cells may spread to choroid and even involve the retina (posterior uveitis). A few patients with AS may have persistent inflammation beyond 3 months (chronic uveitis), especially if they have associated IBD, psoriasis, or reactive arthritis. Rare cases of retinal vasculitis have been reported. These severe forms of uveitis requires more aggressive treatment with monoclonal TNF-inhibitors or even more effective immunosuppressant therapy. Placement of corticosteroid in the outer layers of the eyeball that provides slow release of this medicine for many months is sometimes used. but it markedly increases the risk of cataract (progressive cloudiness and opacity of the lens of the eye).

Possible complications of uveitis

If left untreated or treated inadequately, uveitis may cause permanent impairment of eyesight. Complications from inadequate management, especially of severe recurrent or posterior uveitis, include an elevation of pressure in the eye (glaucoma) that can occur due to adhesion of inflamed iris to its adjacent structures with resultant fixed and/or misshaped pupil. It requires treatment to normalize the pressure because it can lead to a progressive loss of field of vision due to damage to the optic nerve. Some patients need laser surgery to restore normal circulation of fluid in the eye. Some patients may develop cataract that causes glare and reduced vision. It can result from uncontrolled and/or recurrent inflammation, or after chronic use of corticosteroids. Such patients may need surgical lens replacement. Still another but uncommon complication is fluid leakage ("waterlogging") in the central part of the retina (macular edema) that can be easily detected with special new technique called Optical Coherence Tomography (OCT). Rare cases of retinal vasculitis, that is detected by a procedure called fluorescein angiography, can lead to impaired vision due to damage of the retina if it is not recognized and treated aggressively.

7

Other manifestations

 Key points

- People living with AS/axSpA can have inflammation of extra-skeletal sites, such as the eye (discussed in Chapter 6), skin, and intestine (bowel), at some stage during the course of their illness.

- Approximately 10% of patients suffer from psoriasis and 6% have symptoms resulting from inflammatory bowel disease (IBD), discussed in Chapter 10. This chapter deals with the less common involvements of the lungs, heart, kidneys, and the nervous system.

- At the more advanced disease stage, patients can develop functional lung impairment because of diminished chest expansion. Some patients may show mild scarring (fibrosis) of the lungs, particularly at its uppermost parts (apical fibrosis). Smoking should be strictly avoided by all patients.

- Heart may rarely develop a slowly progressive fibrosis of the aortic valve, sometimes in association with dilatation of the adjacent aorta, resulting in leaky aortic valve (aortic incompetence). Impairment of the heart's electric conduction system (heart block) can also occur.

- Other rare occurrences discussed in this chapter involve the kidneys and the spinal cord. Post traumatic spinal fractures and resultant surgical fusion in elderly patients carries substantial in-hospital morbidity and mortality.

Introduction

Patients with AS/axSpA have symptoms resulting from inflammation of the musculoskeletal system (the spine, limb joints, and related tissues), but they can also develop inflammation in other parts of the body (the extra-articular symptoms) at some stage during the course of their illness. The most common of them is

Ankylosing Spondylitis and Axial Spondyloarthritis, Second Edition. Muhammad Asim Khan, Oxford University Press.
© Oxford University Press 2023. DOI: 10.1093/oso/9780198864158.003.0007

acute anterior uveitis, as discussed in Chapter 6. Patients should also be carefully evaluated for symptoms and signs arising from inflammation affecting some of the gut for inflammatory bowel disease (IBD) and the skin for psoriasis, discussed in Chapter 10. This chapter deals with the less common involvements of the lungs, heart, kidney, and the nervous system.

Lung

People with AS can complain of pain in their rib cage and it is worsened on coughing or sneezing because of inflammation of the joints where the ribs attach to the backbone. Approximately 15% of patients may also complain of anterior chest wall pain and soreness (tenderness) due to inflammation at the junction of breast bones (sternum and manubrium) or where they attach to the collar bones (clavicles) and the ribs (costochondral junction).

At the more advanced disease stage, patients can develop functional lung impairment because of restricted chest expansion resulting from progressive fusion of the ribs with the backbone. However, this does not usually result in breathing insufficiency because of compensatory increased use of diaphragm muscles (that separates the lungs from the abdomen) used in normal breathing. Some of the patients may take longer to recover from bronchitis and viral or bacterial lung infections. Patients should therefore be encouraged to get vaccinated against viral infections and bacterial pneumonia. Smoking cigarettes/cigars, including electronic cigarettes (e-cigarettes), should be completely avoided by all patients because it is also associated with impaired response to treatment and leads to worse disease outcomes.

Some patients may show mild changes (fibrosis) in the lungs that is only detected by high-resolution CT scan. On rare occasions patients with long-standing AS can show worsening fibrosis at the uppermost parts (apical fibrosis) of the lung and, rarely, small cavitations and secondary infections.

More recently an association with obstructive sleep apnea has been reported, especially among those with rigid and stooped neck, or who are markedly overweight or obese. These patients may require use of breathing assistance (continuous positive airways pressure [CPAP] or bilevel positive airways pressure [BiPAP]) machines at night for better sleep.

Heart

Some patients have impaired relaxation of their heart muscle (diastolic dysfunction) but with normal ability to contract to pump blood out. There is an uncommon occurrence of a slowly progressive inflammation and resultant scarring (fibrosis) at the root of the aorta (where it comes off from the heart) after many years of the disease. This inflammation (aortitis) can extend to the adjacent initial few centimeters of the wall of the aorta and can be much better visualized by positron emission tomography (PET)/CT imaging. This aortitis can lead to weakness and resultant dilatation (ballooning) of the aortic wall and even impair proper closing of the valve and causing it to leak (aortic valve insufficiency), which can easily be detected by ultrasound study of the heart (echocardiography). It can also occur due to scarring of the valve leaflets independent of adjacent aortitis.

Aortic valve insufficiency or incompetence can lead to heart failure with resultant leg or ankle swelling (edema) and shortness of breath during exertion or exercise. Therefore, it requires regular monitoring and some patients undergo aortic valve replacement by a noninvasive or surgical procedure. Impairment of electric conduction system of the heart can also occur that can lead to irregular and slow heartbeat (pulse) that may become serious enough for some patients to require implantation (under the skin) of a cardiac (heart) pacemaker.

The risk for aortic insufficiency and electric conduction disturbances increases with the age of the patient, the duration of AS, the presence of HLA-B27, and limb joints involvement. Thus, electric conduction disturbances occur in up to 3% of those with disease of 15 years' duration and up to 9% after 30 years. Very rarely, aortic valve insufficiency may have a more rapid course in relatively young patients with minimal spondylitis.

Lastly, it is worth stating that, as among the general population, high blood pressure, high blood cholesterol, smoking, and sedentary lifestyle increases the risk of coronary (heart) artery disease and stroke.

Kidney

Kidney disease in AS can occur for various reasons and present with protein leakage in the urine, sometimes associated with presence of red cells, detected on routine urinalysis, with or without impairment of kidney function. NSAIDs can cause fluid retention, mostly manifested by swelling of the ankles. Their long-term use can impair the normal functioning of the kidneys and can also cause hypertension (increased blood pressure) or blunt the effect of drugs used to treat it, such as diuretics (water pills), angiotensin-converting-enzyme (ACE) inhibitors (such as lisinopril), and ACE-receptor blockers (such as losartan). This makes the chronic use of NSAIDs risky for patients who already have any form of kidney disease, and for the elderly population. NSAIDs can also, on rare occasions, cause acute inflammation in the kidneys, called acute interstitial nephritis, after a few days of use.

Nephritis (kidney inflammation) can also result from deposition of an im-munoglobulin (Ig) protein called IgA and resulting in leakage of protein and blood cells in the urine, with or without impairment of kidney function. It is frequently under-recognized. and is mostly reported from Asian countries. Deposition in the kidneys of another protein called amyloid (amyloidosis) has now become very rare in economically developed countries due to very ef-fective management of AS and is now mainly seen in non-compliant patients with poorly controlled disease.

Neurological problems

Neurologic involvement may occur in patients with AS due to post-traumatic fracture of the spinal column, and any resultant spinal fusion surgery can have serious in-hospital complications. Unstable spinal fracture can increase the risk of spinal cord injury that can result in unfavorable outcome and even paraplegia, or quadriplegia in case of neck fracture. A recent study from the US of 8,526 AS patients who underwent spinal fusion surgery for their spinal fractures (that were equally divided between cervical (neck) versus thoraco-lumbar regions), reported that elderly patients (≥70 years of age) had higher in-hospital complications compared to those who were <70 years of age (57% versus 38%). Also 9.9% of elderly patients had in-hospital mortality compared to 3.1% of younger patients.

There is also a rare and very slowly progressive complication in patients with very long-standing severe AS. It is called *cauda equina* (meaning horsetail) *syn-drome* because of the involvement of lowermost spinal nerves that slope down-ward as a bunch (looking like a horsetail) before leaving the spinal column. This condition results from slowly progressive fibrous entrapment and scar-ring of these nerve roots, and that can result in "saddle anesthesia" (so-called because of loss of skin sensation over the parts we sit on). It can also lead to decreased urinary sphincter and rectal tone with resultant urinary and fecal incontinence. Men may develop erectile dysfunction or impotence. It may also cause some pain and weakness in the legs. Its characteristic feature is the pres-ence of enlarged sacs containing spinal fluid and erosions of the spinal canal, best seen on a CT or an MRI.

Rare co-occurrences of AS and multiple sclerosis have been reported but an association between the two diseases has not been established. Although TNF-inhibitors are generally well tolerated as a treatment by patients with AS, there have been rare but well-documented reports of peripheral neuropathies, in-cluding Guillain–Barre syndrome, or some manifestations that may resemble atypical multiple sclerosis.

8

Physical examination and laboratory tests

> ## ➡ Key points
>
> ◆ Physical signs are sometimes minimal in the early stages of the disease and therefore the physical examination needs to be comprehensive and include looking for inflamed bony attachment of ligaments (enthesitis).
>
> ◆ Unless the examiner has ample clinical experience, many cases will be missed at this early stage, but early diagnosis and proper medical management are crucial for best outcome.
>
> ◆ The disease course is quite variable among patients. However, the typical limitation of spinal mobility and physical deformities of AS usually evolve within the first 10 years.
>
> ◆ Important predictors of spinal disease progression are baseline presence of bony structural damage in the form of fine bony bridging (syndesmophytes) between adjacent vertebrae visible on X-ray examination, elevated CRP, obesity, male gender, HLA-B27, cigarette smoking, and non-compliance by the patient.
>
> ◆ There is no specific "diagnostic" laboratory marker for AS/axSpA, and the diagnosis is based on clinical history, physical examination, and imaging findings.
>
> ◆ *HLA-B27* is a normal gene present worldwide and testing for its presence has demonstrated clinical utility in recognizing AS and related forms of SpA in certain clinical situations.

Ankylosing Spondylitis and Axial Spondyloarthritis, Second Edition. Muhammad Asim Khan, Oxford University Press.
© Oxford University Press 2023. DOI: 10.1093/oso/9780198864158.003.0008

Introduction

Physical signs are sometimes minimal in the early stages of the disease and the physical examination needs to be comprehensive so as not to overlook early physical findings. The examiner should search for signs of soreness (tenderness) where ligaments and tendons attach to the bone (enthesis) in the feet and along the spine. Clinical signs related to inflamed enthesis, called *enthesitis*, are present in many patients but are often overlooked. Therefore, a comprehensive examination includes looking for tenderness over the vertebral spinal processes in the mid-line in the back (spine), bony rim of the pelvis (iliac crest), anterior chest wall (breastbone and adjacent ribs), heel bone (plantar fasciitis), Achilles' tendon insertion at the back of the heel, kneecap (patella) and the bony prominence below it (the tibial tubercle). Inflammation can also affect structures adjacent to the joints, such as tendons and bursa, resulting in tendonitis and bursitis.

Figure 8.1 illustrates most of the physical findings of AS. Pain may be elicited on firm direct pressure one or both SI joint area, usually the first site of inflammation, or on stress-testing them by certain maneuvers (Figure 8.1 h and i). The ability to bend the spine backwards and sideways (without bending the knees), and to rotate the spine, are generally the first to be impaired (Figures 8.1 a, c, d, e). Many patients with good mobility in their hip joints can bend forward quite well, and even touch the ground with their fingertips (Figure 8.1 b). However, a careful examination of lumbar spinal mobility will often detect a decrease in the forward-bending flexibility of this part of their spine. This can be done by performing the Schober test in which the distance between two marks on the lumbar spine 10 cm apart in the mid-line should stretch at least to 12.5 cm (Figure 8.1 g).

Neck rotation (by asking the patient to look over their shoulder) and forward and upward bending should be checked. The doctor should also check for any restriction of chest expansion and examine limbs for any signs of joint inflammation and restricted range of motion, especially of the hip and shoulder joints which are affected in one-third of patients. Chest expansion is measured by a tape measure placed around the chest at nipple level (below the breasts in females) and noting the difference in measurements after full inspiration (breathing in) and full expiration (breathing out). Any forward stooping of the neck can be quantified by having the patients stand erect with the back against a wall, heels touching the wall, and knees fully stretched, and then measuring distance between back of the head (occiput) and the wall (Figure 8.1 f). It is called "occiput-to-wall" test.

Hip joint involvement is usually bilateral and insidious in onset; the pain is usually felt in the groin. Some degree of contracture of the hip joints is not

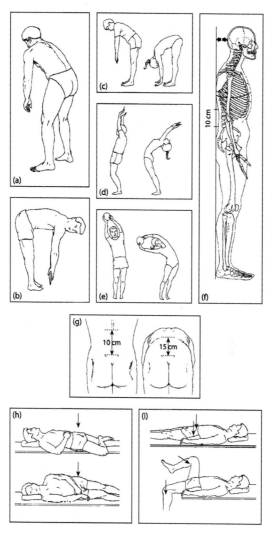

Figure 8.1 It depicts various components of physical examination by healthcare providers, showing limitation of spinal mobility on forward flection (Figures a, b, and c), hyperextension (d), and lateral flexion (e). Measurement of forward stooping of the neck (f) that can be quantitated by measuring occiput (back of the head) to wall distance, while Figure (g) shows measurement of limitation of mobility of the lower back (lumbar spine). Finally, Figures (h) and (i) show assessment of any accentuation of pain on stressing the sacroiliac joints, and degree of flection of the hip joints. (Note: Figures c, d, and e of an AS patient and his physical therapist were drawn from photographs provided by Heinz Baumberger, PhD.)

uncommon at later stages of the disease, giving rise to a characteristic rigid gait, with the patient keeping the knees bent a little to maintain an erect posture. Involvement of peripheral limb joints (other than the hips and shoulder joints) is uncommon and is rarely persistent or destructive, unless it is associated with IBD or psoriasis. The examiner should also check for current or residual signs of eye inflammation, and some patients can have dry eyes.

The disease course and outcomes are quite variable in early stages; the typical limitation of spinal mobility and physical deformities usually evolve within 10 years. Important predictors of spinal disease progression are baseline presence of bony structural damage in the form of fine bony bridging (syndesmophytes) between adjacent vertebrae, elevated CRP (implying persistent inflammation), obesity, males gender, HLA-B27, cigarette smoking, and non-compliance with the recommended treatment. *Syndesmophytes* are vertically orientated ligamentous bone deposits (ossification) producing fine bony bridging between adjacent vertebral bodies at the margin of the vertebrae, characteristic of AS (Figure 8.2 and Figure 8.3).

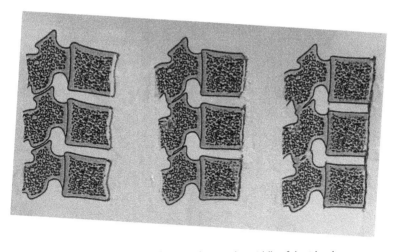

Figure 8.2 A simplified drawing of a vertical cut in the middle of the 3 lumbar vertebrae that shows, from left to right, progressive "squaring" and fusion of the vertebral bodies in the front due to bony bridging (syndesmophytes) and accompanied by osteoporosis and gentle anterior stooping of the spine. There is also progressive narrowing and ultimate fusion of the facet joints that form the back components of the bodies of the vertebra. These facet joints assist in spinal rotation, especially in the neck. The mottled area represents the bone marrow.

Adapted with permission from Khan MA. "Spondyloarthropathies" in Hunder G (ed), *Atlas of Rheumatology*. Philadelphia, PA: Current Medicine Philadelphia, 2005, 151–80.

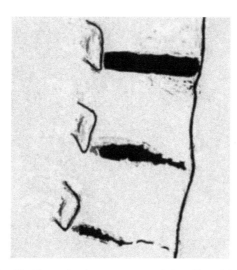

Figure 8.3 A simplified figure showing progressive ankylosis (fusion) between 1st to 3rd lumbar vertebral bodies, as seen from the side; their front surface is facing to the right side. There is progressive bony fusion by syndesmophytes surrounding and partially hiding the lower two inter-vertebral discs. An X-ray can reveal that the discs between the vertebral bodies retain their normal structure and height (unlike the degenerative disc disease), but they may sometimes transform into bone at very late stage (as shown in Figure 26.1).

However, in some patients the disease may remain limited to the SI joints, and spinal fusion (ankylosis) may not occur at all. But in most patients, the disease is progressive, and among those with severe disease there can be gradual forward stooping of the spine and flattening of the anterior chest wall, accompanied by "stooped" shoulders, protuberant abdomen, and breathing becomes increasingly diaphragmatic (Figure 8.4). Spinal ankylosis may progress more slowly in women than in men, but functional outcome, as analyzed by studying activities of daily living, is similar. Neurologic complications of AS are uncommon and mostly result from spinal cord injury due to spinal fracture. With longer disease duration and disease progression, the entire spine can fuse (ankylose), including the cervical spine, along with a gradual development of worsening spinal posture.

Laboratory findings

There is no specific "diagnostic" laboratory marker for AS/axSpA, and the diagnosis is based on clinical history, physical examination, and imaging findings. Acute phase reactants such as elevated CRP and ESR are often used as part

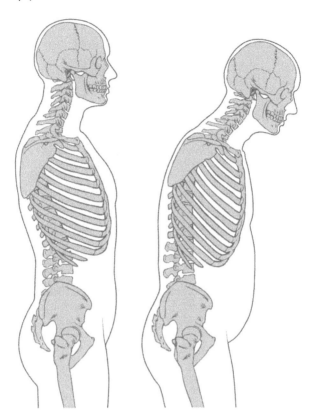

Figure 8.4 Drawings depicting a lateral view of a patient before (left) and after suffering from AS for quite a few years (right), which has resulted in a completely fused spine. Notice the forward stooping of the neck, "flattening" of the anterior chest, prominence of the abdomen, mild flexion contractures of the hip joints, and a loss of body height.

Adapted with permission from Khan MA. "Spondyloarthropathies" in Hunder G (ed), *Atlas of Rheumatology*. Philadelphia, PA: Current Medicine Philadelphia, 2005, 151–80.

of the laboratory work-up of inflammatory rheumatic diseases, but they are elevated in approximately 50% of patients, often those with peripheral arthritis and spinal involvement. Thus, normal values do not exclude the presence of clinically active AS. Measurement of CRP is preferred over ESR for clinical assessment and follow-up. There is no association with rheumatoid factor and antinuclear antibodies, and the synovial fluid and synovial biopsy do not show markedly distinctive features compared with other inflammatory forms of

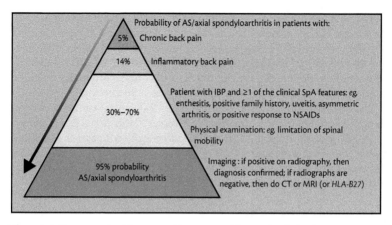

Figure 8.5 Shows an algorithm comprising sequential steps that help clinicians in making an early diagnosis of AS/axSpA with increasing levels of confidence from approximately 5% starting at the top of the pyramid to 95% at the base of the pyramid, based on additional features exhibited by the patient. It does require exclusion of disease mimickers (look-alike diseases).

Adapted with permission from Khan MA. "Spondyloarthropathies" in Hunder G (ed), *Atlas of Rheumatology*. Philadelphia, PA: Current Medicine Philadelphia, 2005, 151–80.

arthritis. Stool examination and consultation with a gastroenterologist may be of value in patients with bowel symptoms to look for concomitant IBD. When reactive arthritis is suspected on clinical grounds, bacterial studies might provide helpful information in some instances.

Figure 8.5 shows probability-based diagnosis algorithm (sequential steps) that helps experienced clinicians make an early diagnosis of AS/axSpA. The term CT in this figure implies the use of low-dose CT that is becoming more widely available and results in much lower exposure to radiation than the standard CT.

HLA-B27 test

It is a relatively inexpensive test that does not need to be repeated (unless for technical/laboratory error), and is discussed in detail in Chapter 3. It does not provide much help in differentiation among the different forms of SpA and cannot be thought of as a routine, diagnostic, confirmatory, or screening test for AS/axSpA in patients presenting with back pain or arthritis. In such patients, if the clinical history and physical examination do not suggest AS, testing for HLA-B27 will be inappropriate because a positive result would still not permit the diagnosis of AS to be made.

However, it has demonstrated clinical utility in recognizing AS/axSpA or related forms of SpA in certain clinical situations. For example, if the history and physical examination findings suggest AS/axSpA but the X-ray or MRI findings do not permit this diagnosis to be made, presence of HLA-B27 markedly enhances this likelihood. Defining the HLA-B27-positive population in the general population has little practical value because no effective means of prevention are currently available, and most (~ 95%) of them will never develop these diseases. However, as discussed in Chapter 3, this risk is higher among HLA-B27-positive children of HLA-B27-positive affected parents. HLA-B27 typing of patients with uveitis helps ophthalmologists in referring patients for rheumatology consultation, especially those with associated back pain or other symptoms that suggest presence of AS/axSpA.

9

Radiology, MRI, and CT

 Key points

◆ All forms of musculoskeletal imaging have a possible role in the work-up of patients with various forms of SpA. Evidence of inflammation and/or structural damage of the SI joint (sacroiliitis) is one of the hallmarks of AS/axSpA.

◆ Obtaining the plane anterior–posterior (AP) pelvic X-ray (or an angled Ferguson's view) is the first step to look for structural damage of the SI joints (sacroiliitis).

◆ However, such an X-ray can sometimes be normal or may be difficult to interpret due to various reasons, particularly among patients seen at a very early stages of their disease.

◆ In this situation, an MRI scan appears to be the method of choice for early detection of sacroiliitis. Moreover, it is radiation-free, although it takes more time, is much more costly, and may be unavailable in some parts of the world.

◆ Low-dose CT can better detect structural damage with minimal radiation, and three-dimensional (3D) reconstruction can help in planning surgical procedures.

◆ Ultrasound examination with high-frequency color and power Doppler can be helpful for evaluating peripheral arthritis, tendinitis, and enthesitis. Ultrasonography can also be helpful in correctly placing the needle to aspirate joint fluid or for joint injection.

Introduction

All forms of musculoskeletal imaging have a possible role in the work-up of patients with SpA. Evidence of involvement (inflammation and/or structural damage) of the SI joint (sacroiliitis) is one of the hallmarks of AS/axSpA.

Ankylosing Spondylitis and Axial Spondyloarthritis, Second Edition. Muhammad Asim Khan, Oxford University Press.
© Oxford University Press 2023. DOI: 10.1093/oso/9780198864158.003.0009

However, it may be difficult to determine, especially in the early stages of the disease, because the SI joints are deep and almost motionless, and there may be no obvious tenderness on direct pressure over the joint. A presumptive clinical diagnosis of AS/axSpA (in the presence of suggestive clinical history) can be confirmed by musculoskeletal imaging.

Radiography

Finding the characteristic changes on an X-ray (bone erosions, narrowing or fusion of the SI joints) that result from inflammatory involvement and any resultant damage are usually present by the time patients seek medical attention. Moreover, these X-ray abnormalities are helpful in distinguishing it from other diseases (differential diagnosis) discussed in Chapter 10.

Radiographic (X-ray) evidence of erosions typical of sacroiliitis is the most consistent and characteristic feature of AS (Figure 1.4); it is usually bilateral and symmetrical and typically first involves the lower ventral (synovial) part of the SI joints (Figure 1.5). Radiography can also detect progressive bony fusion of the SI joints and the spine in later stages of the disease.

Obtaining the conventional anterior–posterior view ("AP view") or an "angled" (Ferguson) views of the pelvis on X-ray is the first and usually sufficient step to look for sacroiliitis as part of AS/axSpA. However, interpretation of radiographs of the SI joints can often be quite challenging even among experienced readers for various reasons. The SI joint has several unique anatomic features and marked variability of its shape in the general population. This makes it difficult to profile the SI joints well on an AP view.

The X-ray can be normal or show only equivocal (unclear) changes in very early stages of the disease (when the structural changes in the joint are still mostly limited to the joint lining (synovial membrane) and the cartilage and have not yet eroded the underlying bone). Oblique views of the individual SI joints are not advised as they are associated with excessive gonadal (testes and ovaries) radiation, while a posteroanterior (PA) view can be useful although usually not needed. Therefore, in certain cases, such as young patients and those with short symptoms, MRI of the SI joints can be an alternative first step.

Magnetic resonance imaging (MRI)

Magnetic resonance

Because the onset of the disease is usually preceded by a long latent period and an early diagnosis is needed to ensure proper and timely treatment, safe and better techniques are needed to detect sacroiliitis accurately. In a situation where pelvic X-ray is normal or unclear but the clinical suspicion of axSpA remains high, an MRI scan of the SI joints is recommended for the early detection of inflammation in the SI joints because conventional radiography only visualizes the late structural consequences of the inflammatory process. MRI can detect both active inflammatory changes (primarily bone-marrow edema) and structural lesion (such as bone erosions and new bone formation). Moreover, unlike radiography, MRI uses no ionizing radiation and is therefore a useful tool, especially in young people, but it is much more costly and may not be available in some parts of the world.

Combination of the MRI of the SI joints with that of the spine adds little incremental value for recognizing patients with early axSpA. Therefore, MRI of the spine is generally not recommended, but it may detect spinal inflammation in some patients with nr-axSpA and juvenile or related SpA. MRI can also be used for early detection of inflammation at other sites by getting a "whole-body MRI" scan that can show widespread sites of inflammation. It may be of benefit for predicting radiographic progression of AS because involvement of the spinal junction of ribs (costovertebral and costotransverse joints) markedly increases the risk for radiographic progression in a subgroup of patients with normal X-ray of their spine.

Low dose computed tomography (CT)

CT may provide more clear information on structural bone damage if conventional radiography is negative, and MRI is unavailable or cannot be performed. CT provides exact depiction of the bones, and 3D reconstructions can also be performed that can be helpful in planning surgical procedures. However, CT is associated with excessive radiation and therefore CT with minimal radiation (low-dose CT) has been developed that has enhanced its clinical utility. When spinal fracture is suspected, conventional radiography is the recommended initial imaging method and if it is negative, CT with minimal radiation dose should be performed. MRI can provide added information on soft tissue lesions.

Ultrasonography

When inflammation is clinically suspected in the limb joints, tendons, and bony attachments of ligament, ultrasonography with high-frequency color or power Doppler can provide additional findings that may support the diagnosis of SpA. Ultrasonography can be helpful in placing the needle in the joint or tendon sheath to aspirate joint fluid or for local injection of medications. Lastly, bone scintigraphy ("bone scan") is not helpful for the diagnosis of AS/axSpA.

10

Diagnosis and management of other forms of SpA and "look-alikes"

 Key points

◆ People suffering from IBD, psoriasis, acute anterior uveitis, or reactive arthritis have increased risk of developing of SpA, either its axial form (AS/axSpA) or peripheral SpA.

◆ Thus, up to 30% of people with psoriasis develop psoriatic arthritis, a form of SpA, and 5–20% of people with CD and, less often, those suffering from ulcerative colitis (UC) develop SpA.

◆ The reverse is also true: patients with SpA are more likely than the general population to also suffer from IBD, psoriasis, acute anterior uveitis, or reactive arthritis. Thus, asymptomatic IBD may be present in close to 60% of all patients with AS, and 5–20% develop CD within the first 5 years of AS presentation.

◆ Luckily, patients with these various forms of SpA respond very well, with very few exceptions, to many of the currently available biologics, especially monoclonal TNF inhibitors and/or tsDMARDs.

◆ This chapter discusses the various forms of SpA and also their differentiation from each other and from other diseases ('look-alikes"), such as diffuse idiopathic skeletal hyperostosis (DISH).

Ankylosing Spondylitis and Axial Spondyloarthritis, Second Edition. Muhammad Asim Khan, Oxford University Press.
© Oxford University Press 2023. DOI: 10.1093/oso/9780198864158.003.0010

Introduction

There are various forms of SpA that include AS and their symptoms usually begin in the late teens and early twenties, but they can also begin in childhood or later in life. They show a strong association with HLA-B27 but the strength of this association varies markedly, not only between the various forms of SpA but also among racial and ethnic groups. Their mode of presentation is also quite varied and, except for AS, may not necessarily develop sacroiliitis or spondylitis. It may also not be always possible to differentiate clearly between the various forms, especially in their early stages, because they generally share many clinical features, both skeletal and extra-skeletal.

Forms of SpA

Besides AS, the various other forms of SpA are divided into:

- Psoriatic arthritis that occurs in association with psoriasis

- Enteropathic SpA occurring in association with IBD

- Reactive arthritis (Reiter's syndrome)

- Juvenile SpA: a form of juvenile chronic arthritis

- Undifferentiated SpA

Patients with psoriasis, IBD, or reactive arthritis are more likely to develop AS than the rest of the population. The reverse is also true; that is, patients with AS are more likely than the general population to suffer from IBD, psoriasis, or reactive arthritis as well as their AS. Moreover, the clinical features typical of SpA may occur in different combinations, so the above-mentioned disease classification may not be appropriate for some patients. The European Spondyloarthropathy Study Group (ESSG) developed classification criteria (Table 10.1) in 1991 to include this currently recognized wider spectrum of SpA. Then in 2009 the Assessment of SpondyloArthritis international Society (ASAS) developed criteria for axSpA (Table 10.2).

Please note that the classification criteria discussed in this chapter were developed by "SpA experts" to select from among the already diagnosed patients a homogeneous subset for participation in clinical research and drug trials. They are not meant to be used for diagnosing an individual patient in clinical practice because they do not contain exclusions of other conditions (look-alikes or disease-mimickers) that is required for a diagnosis.

Table 10.1 The European SpA Study Group (ESSG) criteria for classifying disease as a SpA. Please note that the classification criteria are applied to patients with an established diagnosis to define a group of SpA patients for research. They are no diagnostic criteria that are needed for a clinician to estimate the likelihood of suspected SpA in an individual patient.

SpA is defined as the presence of **inflammatory spinal pain** or **synovitis** *and* **one or more of the following:**

- **family history:** presence, in first- or second-degree relatives, of: ankylosing spondylitis, psoriasis, acute iritis, reactive arthritis, or inflammatory bowel disease.
- **psoriasis**
- **inflammatory bowel disease**
- **alternating buttock pain**
- **enthesitis**
- **acute diarrhea**
- **urethritis**
- **sacroiliitis:** bilateral grade 2–4 or unilateral grade 3–4

Definitions used in these criteria

Inflammatory spinal pain: history of or current symptoms of spinal pain (low, mid, and upper back, or neck region), with at least 4 of the following five components:

  a. at least 3-months duration

  b. onset before age 45

  c. insidious (gradual) onset

  d. improved by exercise

  e. associated with morning spinal stiffness

Synovitis: past or present asymmetric arthritis, or arthritis predominately in the lower limbs
Psoriasis: past or present psoriasis diagnosed by a doctor
Inflammatory bowel disease: past or present UC or CD diagnosed by a doctor and confirmed by radiographic examination or endoscopy
Alternating buttock pain: past or present pain alternating between the two buttock regions
Enthesitis: past or present spontaneous pain or tenderness at examination of the site of the insertion of the Achilles tendon or plantar fascia
Acute diarrhea: episode of diarrhea occurring within 1 month before arthritis onset
Urethritis: nongonococcal urethritis or cervicitis occurring within 1 month before arthritis onset
Sacroiliitis grading system: 0 = normal, 1 = possible, 2 = minimal, 3 = moderate, 4 = completely fused (ankylosed).

Source: data from Amor B, Dougados M, and Mijiyawa M. "Criteria of the classification of spondylarthropathies" [in French]. *Rev Rhum Mal Osteoartic.* 1990;57:85–9.

Table 10.2 The Assessment of Axial Spondyloarthritis international Society (ASAS) classification criteria for axial SpA. As noted earlier, these classification criteria are applied to patients with an established diagnosis of axSpA to define a group of patients for research. There are currently no diagnostic criteria for axSpA that are needed for the clinician to estimate the likelihood of suspected axSpA in an individual patient.

Patients With Back Pain ≥3 Months and Age at Onset <45 Years		
Sacroiliitis on Imaging Plus ≥1 SpA Feature	*or*	HLA-B27 Plus ≥2 Other SpA Features
Sacroiliitis on Imaging • Active (acute) inflammation on MRI highly suggestive of sacroiliitis associated with SpA OR • Definite radiographic sacroiliitis according to modified New York criteria		*SpA Features* • Inflammatory back pain • Arthritis • Enthesitis (heel) • Uveitis • Dactylitis • Psoriasis • CD/UC • Good response to NSAIDs • Family history for SpA • HLA-B27 • Elevated CRP

Reproduced with permission from Rudwaleit M, van der Heijde D, Landewé R, *et al.* "The development of Assessment in SpondyloArthritis International Society (ASAS) classification criteria for axial spondyloarthritis (Part II): Validation and final selection" *Ann Rheum Dis.* 2009; 68(6):777–83.

Psoriatic arthritis

Psoriatic arthritis (abbreviated as PsA) is a type of inflammatory arthritis that occurs among some people with psoriasis, a non-contagious chronic skin and nail disease that is more prevalent in populations of European ancestry than in Asians, Africans, and native Americans. More than 7 million people in the US live with this psoriasis. It results from an abnormal proliferation of skin cells (called *keratinocytes*), induced by T lymphocytes, but the precise cause is not yet fully understood. A family history of psoriasis or PsA is present in up to 40% of patients, and genetic studies suggest that several genes are involved (a *multigenic* mode of inheritance).

There are 5 different types of psoriasis, and the most common (~ 85%) among them is called plaque psoriasis that causes circumscribed patches of slightly raised pink or red skin among people with very light skin complexion but has darker color among others based on their skin pigment. The rash can be itchy and painful and is often covered with silvery or white dry scales that fall off easily when scratched. These are often located over the elbows, knees, scalp, ears, and back. The nails of fingers and toes are affected in more than 80% of patients in the form of pitting, ridging, discoloration, and thickening of the skin under the nails. Sometimes there can be loosening and even loss of the affected nail.

Clinical features

It is estimated that ~ 30% of people with psoriasis develop PsA that affects men and women equally and it usually begins between 30 and 50 years of age, although it can begin in childhood. Even a mild degree of psoriasis can be associated with severe PsA. Among ~ 85% of patients, the arthritis develops after skin psoriasis, usually 5 to 7 years after the appearance of skin disease. Among the rest of the patients the arthritis may precede the onset or the diagnosis of psoriasis, or the two may have almost a simultaneous onset. More than 50% of patients wait for over two years for a diagnosis.

Patients complain of painful swelling and stiffness in one or more small and/or large joints that feel warm and tender to touch. Painful diffuse swelling and stiffness of the fingers and toes is one of the quite characteristic signs of PsA. It is called "*dactylitis*" (from the Greek word "*dactylos*," which means finger (digit). It has also earned the nickname "sausage digits" because of their diffuse swelling of fingers or toes, often associated with involvement of the nails. There is also inflammation at bony sites of attachment of ligaments and tendons called *entheses*, resulting in enthesitis. Thus, enthesitis in the ankle, can cause swelling and tenderness in the back of the foot (*Achilles' tendinitis*) and inflammation of ligaments inserted into the heels to support the arch of the foot (*plantar fasciitis*). Therefore, foot pain can be a common complaint of patients with PsA. Some patients may get episodes of conjunctivitis and/or acute iritis, or concomitant IBD.

PsA has been traditionally divided into the following five types since its detailed description in 1970:

◆ inflammatory arthritis, primarily involving the distal small joints of fingers or toes

◆ asymmetric inflammatory arthritis, involving a few of the joints of the limbs

◆ arthritis of the SI joint and the spine (psoriatic SpA)

◆ symmetrical arthritis of multiple joints, resembling rheumatoid arthritis

◆ arthritis mutilans, a very deforming and destructive (mutilating) form

The exact prevalence of each of these forms of PsA is difficult to establish as disease patterns may differ among various population groups and may even change with time in an individual patient, and some may show overlapping features. The symptoms can worsen over time, but one can have periods of remission with hardly any symptoms, especially in very early stages of the disease. The arthritis mutilans form of PsA is now rarely seen in economically developed countries.

The affected joints may show anything from mild to severe erosions and even severe bone destruction and occasionally fusion on X-ray examination. Chronic inflammatory back pain can be present in patients with PsA due to arthritis of the SI joint and the spine. Men show more severe radiographic damage (both axial and peripheral), whereas women have relatively more non-erosive peripheral joint involvement, pain, and impairment of quality of life. X-ray evidence of sacroiliitis occurs in more than 15% of patients and more than 5% develop prominent spondylitis (psoriatic SpA) with disease features lying between AS and typical peripheral PsA; these percentages increase over time, especially among HLA-B27-positive patients and they are also more likely to develop one or more episodes of acute iritis.

The Classification Criteria for Psoriatic Arthritis (CASPAR) criteria that the patient has established inflammatory arthritis and other "look-alikes" have been excluded. These criteria require that the patient must score at least 3 points from the following items:

- Current psoriasis (assigned a score of 2)
- A history of psoriasis (in the absence of current psoriasis (assigned a score of 1))
- A family history of psoriasis but no current psoriasis and history of psoriasis (assigned a score of 1)
- Dactylitis (assigned a score of 1)
- Juxta-articular (adjacent to joint) new-bone formation (assigned a score of 1)
- Negative test for rheumatoid factor (assigned a score of 1)
- Nail involvement (assigned a score of 1)

Management

PsA can be a serious chronic inflammatory condition that can, in severe cases, result in disability and decreased life expectancy of around three years compared to people without this condition. This mainly results from higher burden of comorbid (concurrent) conditions, such as hypertension, diabetes, obesity, high cholesterol, cardiovascular disease, and IBD. These and the other comorbid conditions, such as depression, anxiety, gout, and fibromyalgia, also need proper management.

The good news is that the increasingly effective treatments are becoming available to treat plaque psoriasis and PsA (see Chapters 19 and 20) that have substantially helped improve the quality of life and long-term prognosis. TNF inhibitors are still the preferred first-line therapy for patients with active PsA over IL-17 inhibitors (secukinumab (Cosentyx®) and ixekizumab (Taltz®)), the IL-12/23 inhibitor ustekinumab (Stelara®), and the IL-23 inhibitor guselkumab (Tremfya®), according to a new guideline from the American College of Rheumatology and the National Psoriasis Foundation. Risankizumab (Skyrizi®) is the latest IL-23 inhibitor approved for PsA.

The IL-17 inhibitors may be used instead of TNF inhibitors in PsA patients who have severe plaque psoriasis, or if there are contraindications to use TNF inhibitors, such as recurrent infections or congestive heart failure. An IL-17 inhibitor is preferred over ustekinumab, but the latter may be considered in patients with concomitant IBD. Abatacept (Orencia®) is another biologic that is approved for the treatment of PsA; it selectively modulates function of T cells.

Janus kinase (JAK) inhibitor tofacitinib (Xeljanz®) and upadacitinib (Rinvoq®) are also approved for treating active PsA, as is a phosphodiesterase-4 (PD-4) inhibitor named apremilast (Otezla®) (see Chapters 20). They are taken in a tablet form and may be used instead of a TNF inhibitor because of contraindications, or if the patient's psoriasis and PsA are not severe, or for those who prefer a tablet over an injection. These drugs are grouped under the term *"targeted synthetic DMARDs"* (ts-DMARDs) because they are developed to target a particular molecular structure. Sulfasalazine and ethotrexate are conventional synthetic DMARDs (cs-DMARDs) that are still being used for some patients, although they are less effective than the above-mentioned drugs.

Enteropathic arthritis

The epidemiology of IBD is almost evenly split between ulcerative colitis (UC) and CD, and its prevalence is increasing in Western and newly industrialized countries. Approximately 10% of people with UC and 15–20% of people with CD develop arthritis, called enteropathic arthritis, at some stage during their disease. It takes the form of peripheral joint inflammation usually affecting fewer than 5 and mostly large joints in approximately 60–70% of patients. The joint inflammation correlates with flare-up of the bowel disease, especially in the case of UC. The remaining 30–40% of patients with enteropathic arthritis have axial disease called enteropathic SpA with radiographic evidence of sacroiliitis alone or with classic AS. This form does not fluctuate with bowel disease activity.

Conversely, 5–20% of patients with AS develop clinically obvious CD within the first 5 years of AS presentation. Moreover, asymptomatic IBD may be present in close to 60% of all patients with AS, and long-term follow-up studies suggest that approximately one-third of this subset will eventually develop CD.

Symptoms of CD can include pain in lower abdomen, bloating, nausea, flatulence, diarrhea, vomiting, or bowel obstruction. The patients may also have fatigue, weight loss, mouth ulcers, anemia, and some may develop anal fissures or bleeding. Others may have almost no symptom most of their lives, while some can have persistent and/or severe symptoms that never go away. Noninvasive tests include CT scan and radiation-free alternative called magnetic resonance enterography. Diagnosis can be confirmed by endoscopy (including capsule endoscopy) and possibly mucosal biopsy.

Symptoms of UC include diarrhea, often with blood or mucus, cramping and pain in the abdominal pain, urgency to empty the bowel, rectal pain with or without bleeding, fatigue, and weight loss. Symptoms can fluctuate due to spontaneous remissions and flare-ups and can vary between mild and severe forms. Patients are usually diagnosed in their 30s and colonoscopy and mucosal lining biopsy are needed to confirm the diagnosis.

Management

Many effective drugs are now available to treat CD and UC and need for surgery has markedly decreased. The choice depends on severity of the disease. The first drug choice include 5-aminosalicylates (such as sulfasalazine and mesalamine), short-term use of corticosteroids to treat severe flare-ups, immunosuppressants (such as azathioprine, methotrexate, cyclosporine), JAK-inhibitor (tofacitinib®), or biologics (TNF inhibitors except etanercept, ustekinumab, vedolizumab (Entyvio®), and ozanimod (Zeposia®)). NSAIDs may need to be avoided because they may trigger flare-ups of the underlying IBD.

Reactive arthritis (Reiter's syndrome)

Reactive arthritis is an aseptic inflammatory arthritis that follows an episode of urethritis, cervicitis, or diarrhea, and may also show inflammation at sites other than joints, such as eyes, skin, and mouth. This term encompasses the more restrictive and less commonly used term *Reiter's syndrome*. The joint inflammation is triggered by bacterial infection at a distant site, usually in the gastrointestinal (GI) or genitourinary tract. Although the term *reactive arthritis* implies the presence of a triggering infection, but it is not always possible to find the trigger. If the triggering infection produces no symptoms, its presence may be suggested only by a positive antibody test against such infections.

Depending on the bacterial trigger, reactive arthritis can be more common in men than in women. Table 10.3 lists some of the important bacterial triggers. Genitourinary tract infection with *Chlamydia* is the more commonly recognized initiator in the western societies, but enteric infections with *Shigella*,

Table 10.3 Bacteria that can triggering reactive arthritis

Chlamydia trachomatis
Shigella flexneri
Salmonella (many species)
Yersinia enterocolitica and *Y. pseudotuberculosis*
Campylobacter fetus jejuni
Clostridium difficile

In addition, reactive arthritis not associated with HLA-B27 has also been observed following many other bacterial, viral, and parasitic infections, and in association with intestinal bypass surgery, acne, hidradenitis suppurative (abscesses in the armpit and groin), and cystic fibrosis.

Salmonella, *Yersinia*, or *Campylobacter* are more common triggers in developing countries. Sometimes there is no recognized antecedent infection, or the triggering infection may be asymptomatic.

The prevalence and incidence of *Chlamydia*-induced reactive arthritis has declined since 1985 in Europe and the US, but the post-enteritic form of the disease that affects children and adults, both male and female, including elderly people, may be increasing. After some epidemics of bacterial gastroenteritis or food poisoning (e.g., *Salmonella* enteritis), the incidence of reactive arthritis, or at least some form of musculoskeletal inflammation and pain, can be as high as 20% among HLA-B27-positive individuals in the general population, but the initial episode of reactive arthritis in such epidemics is relatively weakly associated with HLA-B27 (not more than 33% of these patients may possess this gene).

Not everyone who develops a potentially triggering infection will develop arthritis, but genetically susceptible individuals, including presence of the *HLA-B27* gene, increases the risk up to 50-fold. The disease tends to be more severe and more likely to become chronic in people with a triggering infection that is symptomatic and proven by bacterial culture, especially if they are born with the *HLA-B27* gene. The prevalence of reactive arthritis in a population varies with the prevalence of the known bacterial triggering infections, and that of the HLA-B27 in the population.

Clinical features

Chlamydia-induced reactive arthritis is most seen in young promiscuous men in the western developed countries. The clinical picture varies from mild *arthritis* to a severely disabling illness that may render the patient bedridden for a few weeks. Many people have only one episode but in some the disease does recur or persist. The arthritis more frequently involves the lower limbs, with the knees and ankles being most affected, followed by the feet, the upper limbs, and the back. General symptoms such as malaise, fever, and aching muscles (myalgia) may occur, and there may also be pain in the lower back and the buttocks (due to sacroiliitis) that feels worse in the early morning.

The acute arthritis is often associated with genitourinary tract inflammation (urethritis and cervicitis), and/or *conjunctivitis* (commonly known as *pink eye*), which is an inflammation of the delicate outer membrane that lines the inside of the eyelids and the white of the eye. The inflammation is usually mild and bilateral, and you may not even notice it. However, it can cause eye irritation and redness, and sometimes your eyelids may stick together in the morning. Some patients may get acute uveitis (see Chapter 5). *Urethritis*, an inflammation of the urethra (a small tube through which urine passes from the bladder to the outside), can cause difficult or painful urination. It occurs much more commonly in post-chlamydial reactive arthritis and is more frequently symptomatic in men than in women and may sometimes result in slight pus or mucus-like urethral discharge, bladder inflammation (cystitis), lower abdomen pain, and urinary frequency. Sometimes the urethritis symptoms may be quite mild, and the doctor will have to ask about them. Prostatitis (an infection or inflammation of the prostate gland in men) often occurs in conjunction with urethritis. The disease is under-diagnosed in women because their chlamydial infection is often subclinical or asymptomatic and also because doctors rarely do pelvic examinations to look for the presence of cervicitis (inflammation of the cervix, the part of the uterus that protrudes into the vagina). People with *post-enteritic reactive arthritis* often describe a history of fever, abdominal pain, and diarrhea preceding the arthritis by 1–4 weeks, but they may sometimes also have sterile (non-infected) urethritis.

Diagnosis

The diagnosis may sometimes be difficult, as there is no specific diagnostic test. A careful clinical history and physical examination is needed to diagnose this condition. Because there is a delay of several days between the triggering infection and the onset of disease, the patient may not relate the two events together and therefore not mention the previous episode of infection to the doctor. The ESR is often high, but this is also common in other inflammatory diseases. Other tests include examination and cultures of synovial (joint) fluid, stool, and urethral discharge. HLA-B27 association is higher among the population of Western European descent with a wide range (35–70%, compared to 6–8% in the general population when compared with some of the other races racial groups.

Reactive arthritis shares many features with PsA, and sometimes a long period of observation may be needed to reach a correct diagnosis. A skin rash resembling psoriasis may appear on the soles of the feet and palms of the hands. It often heals within a few weeks but may need prescription creams. In a few people small, shallow, painless sores may occur on the tongue or roof of the mouth (palate), but they usually heal in a few days or weeks without any scarring, even without any treatment. Similar sores can sometimes occur on the external genitalia, on the tip (glans) or shaft of the penis or on the scrotum in men, and in the vagina in women. They crust over and heal after a few weeks and are not contagious. *Enthesitis* is also an important feature of reactive arthritis, and patient can have inflamed tendon sheaths resulting in sausage-like swelling of the toes or fingers, but less often than in PsA. The nails may also be affected with pitting and discoloration, the so-called plumber's nails.

Management

In most people the disease can be well-managed with treatment, and the outcome is usually good because it is often self-limiting; in other words it goes away without any residual problems. Other people may have recurrent attacks or have a chronic form of the disease with ongoing joint problems, typically recurring arthritis and tendinitis that may result in stiff joints and weak muscles. Back and neck pain and stiffness due to sacroiliitis and spondylitis may also occur. The spondylitis usually does not lead to the bamboo spine typical of AS. But patients who are HLA-B27-positive are more likely to have chronic course and stiffness, evolve into spondylitis, or be associated with acute uveitis. Such patients usually need treatment with biologics.

Childhood-onset (juvenile) spondyloarthritis

When AS occurs before age 16, it is called juvenile AS (JAS), and symptoms start at pre-teen and teen years. They show a strong association with HLA-B27, just like AS of adult onset. Some children have some but not all the features of AS and are diagnosed as having juvenile SpA. Among all children referred to pediatric rheumatic disease clinics, approximately 20% of the children identified as having a discrete rheumatic disease suffer from juvenile SpA. Approximately 2 of every 1,000 children suffer from JAS or juvenile SpA, and boys are more often affected than girls. This disease is different from juvenile inflammatory arthritis (JIA) of polyarticular type.

Improved guidelines for diagnosing childhood rheumatic diseases have contributed to earlier identification of juvenile SpA. There is often no chronic inflammatory lower-back pain, sacroiliitis, psoriatic skin lesions, or intestinal symptoms, and as discussed later, undifferentiated forms of SpA occur more often during childhood and adolescence than in adulthood. Many patients may show a family history of AS, psoriasis, IBD, or acute anterior uveitis.

Intermittent episodes of pain in the groin, worsened on prolonged sitting, and resultant limping without any previous physical trauma or infection, can be a presenting manifestation in some children. Others may present with soreness at bony attachment of ligaments (enthesitis) at multiple sites. Some may present with the syndrome of enthesitis and arthritis (sometimes called SEA syndrome, which stands for seronegative enthesitis and arthritis). If the enthesitis affects the site of attachment of the patellar tendon to the tibial tubercle (a bony prominence couple of centimeters or so below the kneecap), it can sometimes be confused with a childhood condition called *Osgood–Schlatter's disease*. However, a child with juvenile SpA will frequently also show tenderness at other bony sites due to enthesitis, and not just at the tibial tubercles. Reactive arthritis can also occur in children, usually triggered by enteric infection due to *Shigella, Salmonella,* or *Yersinia,* but the arthritis is relatively less severe than in adults. The juvenile onset of psoriatic arthritis is uncommon but well documented.

At least 50% of these young people reach adulthood with persistent (active) arthritis and need further rheumatological care. Their disease may evolve into JAS with back pain, sacroiliitis, and diminished spinal mobility. A study of such patients in Mexico has found that severe enthesitis in the feet is a very common first presentation of AS in a Mestizo population of mixed genetic ancestry (mostly native Americans with some Spanish admixture).

Undifferentiated spondyloarthritis

The term "undifferentiated" or "unclassified" SpA is used to describe symptoms and signs suggesting SpA in someone who does not meet a clinical definition of AS or a related SpA. They may be suffering from a limited form or early stage of the disease, such as a patient suffering from eye inflammation (uveitis), heel pain, and unilateral swollen knee and ankle, and without psoriasis or IBD. The disease may later progress to AS, or the other forms of SpA, which could be considered as "differentiated" SpA.

The undifferentiated forms can occur relatively more commonly in children. In fact, at least 50% of childhood SpA present in an undifferentiated form at onset. The disease may begin with enthesitis causing pain in the heels and other bony sites, or lower extremity arthritis of 1 (especially knee or ankle) or more joints, mostly in boys between the ages of 9 and 16 years, without any other features. This form of arthritis may precede the back pain by several years.

Less than 1 in 4 of children with AS or other forms of SpA initially present with back pain, stiffness, or restricted motion, or symptoms or signs of sacroiliitis.

This is a notable distinction from adults with AS. When a young child presents with isolated signs referable to an SI joint, possible bacterial infection of this joint is also considered. Sometimes leukemia and other forms of malignancy in children may mimic the clinical presentation of juvenile arthritis, including SpA. X-ray evidence of sacroiliitis is one of the diagnostic hallmarks of axSpA in the adult population. However, it is not easy to detect sacroiliitis by conventional radiography in growing children. MRI is helpful in children and adolescents with clinical features suggestive of a SpA, and it does not involve exposure to radiation. A modified form of MRI can distinguish normal changes due to growth of the child from true inflammatory disease.

Miscellaneous conditions that are "look-alikes" (disease mimickers)

Diffuse idiopathic skeletal hyperostosis (DISH), also called Forestier's disease, can cause excessive new bone formation of the spinal ligaments along the spine (with well-preserved discs) and at some other sites. This can result in a stiff spine that may be confused with AS. It usually occurs in elderly individuals, becoming evident on spinal X-rays after 50 years of age.

Osteitis condensans ilii is characterized by benign increased bone density (sclerosis), adjacent to the lower part and to the sacral side of the SI joint, and its X- ray appearance can be confused with sacroiliitis. It is typically bilateral and triangular in shape, usually self-limiting and often asymptomatic. It is most often seen in young multiparous women and is thought to be due to mechanic stress across the SI joints during pregnancy and the post-partum period.

Paget's disease of the pelvis and spine in advanced stage may cause back pain and be confused with AS. It is also called osteitis deformans and is characterized by accelerated bone turnover, resulting in the involved bone becoming enlarged but weak and fragile. The bone also feels warmer to touch due to increased blood supply. *Scheuermann's disease* of the spine is a non-inflammatory spinal disease that occurs in adolescence and affects the thoracic spine, especially the discs. Often painless, but can result in spinal deformity (scoliosis and kyphosis) during period of bone growth during puberty.

SAPHO syndrome (named for its salient features: synovitis, acne, palmoplantar pustulosis, hyperostosis, and aseptic osteomyelitis) and related conditions grouped under the term *chronic non-infectious osteitis* (CNO) can cause chronic backpain and stiffness due to aseptic bone changes in the SI joints or the spine. Other differential diagnoses include osteoarthritis of the back and sacroiliac joints, *sarcoidosis*, osteomalacia, *hyperparathyroidism* (overacting parathyroid gland), and lymphoma or other malignancies.

11

Other causes of chronic back pain

➲ Key points

- AS/axSpA is an important but relatively uncommon cause of common non-specific chronic back pain and is therefore very often overlooked by the primary healthcare providers.

- Fibromyalgia and chronic pain have been a challenge for the physicians to diagnose and treat. They are characterized by chronic widespread pain; the International Association for the Study of Pain (IASP) has re-defined pain as "an unpleasant sensory and emotional experience associated with, or resembling that associated with, actual or potential tissue damage." The IASP also points out that inability to communicate does not negate the possibility that a person experiences pain.

- Osteoporosis is caused by decrease in the bone mineral density (BMD) and can exist for years without any symptoms, but later results in back pain due to fragile bone with increased risk of spinal and limb fractures.

- Osteomalacia can be mistaken for AS/axSpA and fibromyalgia because it causes widespread pain, including back pain, fatigue, weakness, tenderness over bones, and some resemblances to AS/axSpA on X-ray imaging.

- The spread of *cancer* to the pelvis and the spine, as well as some chronic *spinal infections*, can also present as back pain. A very brief discussion of "long COVID" is also provided.

Discussion about pain

Pain is not merely a sensation limited to signals that travel through the nervous system as a result of tissue damage but can be a disease in and of itself. Once

Ankylosing Spondylitis and Axial Spondyloarthritis, Second Edition. Muhammad Asim Khan, Oxford University Press.
© Oxford University Press 2023. DOI: 10.1093/oso/9780198864158.003.0011

a person develops one chronic pain condition, they seem to be predisposed to develop others because, for example, the brain pathways that drive depression are also linked to the ones that drive chronic pain. In 2020, the IASP has redefined pain (since the 1997 definition) that states that "pain is an unpleasant sensory and emotional experience associated with, or resembling that associated with, actual or potential tissue damage." Moreover, the IASP states that pain is always a personal experience "that is influenced to varying degrees by biological, psychological, and social factors," and "individuals learn the concept of pain through their life experiences" and "verbal description is only one of several behaviors to express pain." It is also emphasized that inability to communicate does not negate the possibility that a person experiences pain.

Chronic back pain

Chronic back pain is defined as persistence of pain beyond 3 months. Although it is the most common presenting symptom of patients with AS/axSpA, non-specific or mechanical back pain (muscle sprain and degenerative disc disease), in its acute and chronic forms, is one of the most common health problems in the general population, resulting from a long list of possible causes. AS/axSpA is an important but relatively uncommon cause of back pain in the general population and is thus very often overlooked by the healthcare providers, as well as others such as chiropractors, orthopedists, physiatrists, and physical therapists. A detailed discussion of the numerous causes of back pain is outside the scope of this book.

The spread of *cancer* to the pelvis and the spine, as well as some chronic *spinal infections*, can also present as back pain. Therefore, your doctor requires organized clinical and imaging strategies for its differential diagnosis, keeping in mind the dictum called "striped horses" ("common things occur commonly; when you hear hoof beats, look for horses, not zebras").

Degenerative disc disease

Clinical back pain related to mechanical degenerative changes in the spine increases with age. It is accelerated by physical and mechanical stress and can take many forms but is often related to degeneration of intervertebral discs and related structures. The central part of these discs in childhood consists of over 85% water, but there is a slow but steady decrease with aging, down to about 60% by the age of 80 years. This results in shrinking and decreased of the disc volume causing narrowing of the disc space and buckling of the surrounding ligaments (annulus fibrosus and spinal ligaments). It can also result in the formation of horizontally projecting bony spurs (osteophytes) at the edges of the spinal vertebral bodies, but they look quite different from syndesmophytes of AS/axSpA.

Fibromyalgia (fibrositis) and chronic pain

Some patients with chronic pain and inflammation due to chronic rheumatic diseases, such as axSpA and rheumatoid arthritis, develop pain amplification due to central nervous system sensitization ("central sensitization") that results in hypersensitivity to stimuli from things that are not typically painful. Their pain persists even when the inflammation is completely resolved due to effective medical management. They also have associated fatigue, emotional and mental distress (anxiety, depression, perceived stress), sleep disturbance, and some complain of "mental fogging" (cognitive difficulties). It is a common disorder that occurs in up to 10% of the population in developed countries in North America and Europe, mostly observed among women between the ages of 25 and 55 years. It can occur without any obvious physical injury or illness, or in a separate area of the body from the original site of tissue damage. People with a family history of fibromyalgia are 8 times more likely to suffer from this condition. Some illnesses resulting from infections (see "long COVID" later in this chapter), physical or emotional events, or prolonged psychological stress may trigger or aggravate their symptoms.

The term *fibromyalgia syndrome* (or *chronic widespread pain syndrome*) is used to lump a group of related, undefined conditions characterized by chronic widespread pain that has been a challenge for the physicians to diagnose and manage. Although fibromyalgia and axSpA are two different conditions, they can sometimes cause diagnostic confusion, especially in women.

Healthcare providers, generally speaking, do not treat people with chronic widespread pain well, even though it is one of the leading causes of disability that is predicted to increase as populations age, but it can be managed by a team of healthcare professionals who specialize in its treatment, with patient education and self-management strategies, sometimes combined with medications.

Chronic back pain can also result from other causes, such as chronic spinal infections, lymphoma, and spread of cancer to the back (metastatic cancer).

Long COVID

This is a term commonly used to describe symptoms that usually occur 3 months following initial recovery from an acute COVID-19 infection or that persist from the initial illness and last for at least 2 months and cannot be explained by an alternative diagnosis. The World Health Organization has renamed it "post COVID-19 condition" and its occurrence is greatest in people between 35 and 69 years old, females, and those living in economically deprived areas. Prominent symptoms include persistent fatigue, breathlessness, cognitive decline (such as attention deficit, word recall, memory recall, "brain fog"), depression, headache, and body aches, and may fluctuate or relapse over time and affect people's daily functioning and their capacity to work. Some of the other symptoms resemble fibromyalgia. The underlying cause is not yet fully understood.

Osteomalacia

It is a bone-thinning disorder resulting from deficiency of vitamin D. It should not be mistaken for osteoporosis, although the two can co-occur. Its most common causes include deficiency of dietary in take of vitamin D, lack of adequate skin exposure to sunlight, dietary deficiency, and chronic kidney failure. It can be mistaken for AS/axSpA because it causes widespread pain, including back pain, fatigue, weakness, tenderness over bones, and some resemblance with that of AS/axSpA X-ray imaging. The childhood form of osteomalacia is called rickets, and both can be easily treated with vitamin D therapy.

Osteoporosis

Bones are not lifeless structures and they change (undergo remodeling) during our life. Osteoporosis occurs when too much bone is removed and not enough is replaced.

More than 30% of patients with AS develop severe spinal ankylosis with worsening spinal osteoporosis. This increases the risk for occurrence of multiple spontaneous vertebral compression fractures without displacement, as discussed in Chapter 22, as well as post-traumatic spinal fractures. People with AS are 5 times more likely to get spinal fractures than the general population, and they may follow a relatively minor trauma, especially in people with long-standing AS that has resulted in a fused spine. They usually affect the lower neck (cervical spine). The pain associated with fractures may be overlooked, or wrongly attributed to exacerbation of AS. The best early clues to spinal fracture may be an acute or unexplained onset of back pain, even in the absence of a history of a fall or physical injury, that is aggravated by movement. There may sometimes be an associated localized spinal tenderness over the site of pain.

Osteoporosis is called a silent disease which may be present for years before it causes any symptoms. It can worsen a forwardly stooped spinal posture.

A woman's risk of hip fracture is equal to her combined risk of breast, uterine, and ovarian cancer. Elderly people have an up to 1 in 5 chances of dying in the year following a hip fracture. Moreover, among those who survive there is 1 in 4 chance that they will require long-term care afterward. Osteoporosis is responsible for more than 1.5 million fractures annually in the US. This figure is rising with the increase of the aging population and is already causing an estimated national direct expenditure (hospitals and nursing homes) in the US of at least $14 billion annually (and rising).

Management of osteoporosis

The most widely used screening tool for osteoporosis involves measuring the BMD using a DXA scan. During this painless, quick, and safe test, a person lies on a padded table as a scanner passes over the body, usually over the hip and spine. DXA can help healthcare providers spot bone loss in people who might otherwise have no symptoms. The test is also useful in tracking the beneficial effects of medications used to manage osteoporosis. An available plain X-ray film of the spine may also provide an opportunistic screening, but only detect relatively advanced stage of osteoporosis. Fully automated techniques are being developed for earlier detection of loss of vertebral BMD from analysis of such X-rays with the use of artificial intelligence (AI), also called "deep learning".

Several treatments can help to prevent loss of bone mass and to improve it, but the first step is to consume foods that provide adequate calcium, the mineral essential for bone strength, and vitamin D. Good dietary sources of vitamin D include eggs, mushrooms, and oily fish, such as salmon. Dietary supplements are needed only for people with poor dietary intake, inadequate sun exposure (because they are housebound, or wear clothing that limits their sun exposure), or suffering from conditions that impair fat absorption from the gut (vitamin D is a fat-soluble vitamin). You should not take supplements simply at the suggestion of friends or family members without first consulting your physician or a dietician. Over-supplementations of vitamin D and of other fat-soluble vitamins A, E, and K should be avoided because they are stored in the body for a long period, and this can result in toxicity. On the other hand, the water-soluble vitamins B and C, when taken in excess, are quickly excreted in the urine.

Treatment recommendations for osteoporosis are often based on an estimate of the person's risk of breaking a bone in the next 10 years, and this is determined by DXA. If the risk is high, treatment includes medication, in addition to modifying risk factors for bone loss, injury, and falls. Early control of inflammation by NSAIDs and inhibitors of TNF and IL-17 help improve bone density.

Drugs called bisphosphonates, such as alendronate (Fosamax®), risedronate (Actonel®), ibandronate (Boniva®), and zoledronic acid (Reclast®) are approved for use; their side effects include nausea, heartburn-like symptoms, and abdominal pain. A rare but very serious complications of long-term treatment with bisphosphonates are bone death (osteonecrosis) in the jawbone with delayed healing, and a crack in the middle of the femur (thigh bone). Persons should have a dental examination before starting these medications, and they should take good care of their teeth, and they should tell their dentist that they are taking these medications. There are additional forms of treatment for osteoporosis, such as treatment with female and male hormones, and parathyroid and parathyroid-like hormones that you can discuss with your physician.

A biologic drug called denosumab (Prolia®), delivered via an injection under the skin every 6 months, produces better bone density results, but it is a more costly treatment. Another biologic called romosozumab (Evenity®) is the newest bone-building medication to treat osteoporosis, and it is given as an injection every month but only for 1 year, followed by other osteoporosis medications. It is important to emphasize the need for a regular follow up with your healthcare provider.

12

Assessment of disease activity and functional impairment

 Key points

- It is important to distinguish symptoms that reflect active disease from symptoms of a mechanical, neurological, or psychological nature before making specific treatment decisions.

- Routine blood test such as CRP and ESR may not correlate very well with disease activity. Therefore, several clinical measures have been developed for this purpose and are discussed in this chapter. They also enable better assessment of response to treatment.

- These include disease activity scores, such as the Bath Ankylosing Spondylitis Disease Activity Index (BASDAI), composite score, such as Ankylosing Spondylitis Disease Activity Score (ASDAS), functional disability scores, such as the Bath Ankylosing Spondylitis Functional Index (BASFI), health-related quality of life scores, such as the Assessment of SpondyloArthritis international Society Health Index (ASAS HI), and criteria for response to therapy, such as the ASAS response criteria.

- An increasing number of rheumatologists are incorporating into their clinical practice the *patient-reported outcome* (PRO) measures (PROM). These are defined as any report that provides the status of patient's health condition that comes directly from the patient.

Ankylosing Spondylitis and Axial Spondyloarthritis, Second Edition. Muhammad Asim Khan, Oxford University Press.
© Oxford University Press 2023. DOI: 10.1093/oso/9780198864158.003.0012

Introduction

It is important to distinguish symptoms that reflect active disease from symptoms of a mechanical or psychological nature before making specific treatment decisions, and several clinical measures have been developed for this purpose. They also enable better assessment of response to treatment. Blood test such as CRP and ESR do not correlate very well with disease activity in many patients with AS/axSpA.

Patient-reported outcome (PRO)

PRO measures (PROM) are defined as any report that provides the status of a patient's health condition that comes directly from the patient. They have been developed to complement blood test results and are discussed in this chapter. You can download the clinical measures for assessment of disease activity and functional impairment from the Axial Spondyloarthritis International Federation's (ASIF) website (<http://www.asif.info>), and <http://www.asas-group.org>, the website of Assessment of Spondyloarthritis international Society (ASAS).

Disease activity and response to therapy

BASDAI was the first and a reliable, easy-to-use, and sensitive-to-change measure that was designed by medical professionals in conjunction with patients. It consists of seeking the patient's response to a self-administered questionnaire that contains 6 questions pertaining to the following 5 major symptoms of AS:

1. Fatigue and/or tiredness you have experienced

2. Axial musculoskeletal pain (in the spine, including neck and pelvis, and hip and shoulder girdles) you have had

3. Pain and/or swelling in other (peripheral) joints

4. Discomfort you have had from any areas tender to touch or pressure

5. Overall *level* of morning stiffness you have had from the time you wake up, and its *duration.*

The patient is asked to give an average score during the *preceding one week* on a numeric 0–10 scale (with 0 being the best and 10 being the worst), or a visual analog scale (VAS) that uses a horizontal line 10 centimeters (cm) in length. Notice that there is 1 question each for the first 4 symptoms, and the fifth question relating to morning stiffness has 2 subcomponents (one for severity and the other for duration). Therefore, to give each symptom equal weighting, the average of the 2 scores relating to morning stiffness is used. The resulting total score of these 5 symptoms can range from 0 to 50, and it is divided by 5 to give a final BASDAI score, which can range from 0 to 10.

Scores of 4 or more suggest suboptimal (inadequate) disease control; these patients may be good candidates for a change in their medical therapy, for treatment with biologic therapies, or for enrollment in clinical trials evaluating new drug therapies directed at AS/axSpA. It is worth mentioning that patients with concomitant fibromyalgia may have a high BASDAI score that may not necessarily reflect the level of inflammation.

ASDAS combines (a) 3 questions from the BASDAI (about back pain, peripheral pain/swelling, and the level and duration of morning stiffness); (b) BASFI (discussed later in this chapter); and (c) acute phase reactant (CRP or ESR). It performs better than the BASDAI score. The ASAS website (<http://www.asas-group.org>) offers calculators for both ASDAS and BASDAI, and also relevant information on classification, diagnosis, outcome assessment, and treatment of SpA.

ASAS response criteria with 20% improvement (ASAS20), 50% improvement (ASAS50), or 70% improvement (ASAS70) are measure of short-term improvement in AS that are designed to be used as summary outcomes measures in clinical trials. The ASAS20 response was developed for clinical trials to document efficacy of NSAIDs, and ASAS40 response is more suitable measure with the advent of better response to TNF inhibitors. Another measure named ASAS5/6 is similar to the ASAS-20, ASAS-50, and ASAS-70 responses, except that it contains two more items: the BASMI score (discussed later in this chapter) and CRP. It is so named since it requires achieving at least a 20% improvement in 5 of its 6 components and absence of deterioration in the potentially remaining sixth domain.

PGA (Patient global assessment): It is measured by the question 'How active was your disease last week?' The patient is asked to answer using a numeric 0–10 scale (with 0 being the best and 10 being the worst). Disease remission is being increasingly regarded as an appropriate therapeutic goal for AS because of the availability of more effective therapies, especially in patients at the early stage of their disease. A state of low disease activity has been suggested empirically, but it needs further development and evaluation for defining a state of "true" disease remission in AS.

RAPID3 (Routine Assessment of Patient Index Data 3) is a pooled index of the 3 patient-reported American College of Rheumatology Rheumatoid

Arthritis Core Data Set measures: function, pain, and patient global estimate of status. Each of these 3 individual measures is scored 0–10, for a total of 30. RAPID3 cumulative score is obtained by adding the scores of the 3 measures. Disease activity is considered to be high if the score is >12, moderate if the score is between 6.1 and 12, low if the score is between 3.1 and 6, and the disease is considered to be in remission when the score is 3 or less. RAPID3 can provide a baseline quantitative value that can be used to monitor quantitatively and document improvement or worsening of over time, with minimal effort of the rheumatologist and staff.

MFI (Multidimensional Fatigue Inventory) is a 20-item self-report instrument to measure fatigue. It covers general, physical, and mental fatigue and reduced motivation/activity.

FACIT (Functional Assessment of Chronic Illness Therapy), fourth version, is a 13-item composite scale that is used to evaluate fatigue. It uses a cross-cultural approach.

Functional disability scores

BASFI is also an easy, reliable, and sensitive-to-change method that assesses the degree of functional disability and coping skills on a 10-cm VAS and comprises 10 questions designed by medical professionals in conjunction with patients. The VAS anchors are labeled "easy" and "impossible." The first 8 questions consider activities related to functional abilities (e.g., putting on socks without help or aids, and looking over the shoulder without turning the body), and the final 2 questions assess the patient's ability to cope with everyday life (doing a full day of activities at home or at work, and doing physically demanding activities, e.g., physiotherapy exercises, gardening, or sports). BASFI scores can range from 0 to 10. Higher scores signify greater functional impairment. Another functional index, the Dougados Functional Index, is less popular.

HAQ (Health Assessments Questionnaire) is a tool to evaluate functional disability that was later modified to a shorter version and later to HAQ Disability Index (HAQ-DI). Patients are asked questions about their abilities to perform 8 functional activities of daily living (ADL): dressing, rising, eating, walking, hygiene, reaching, gripping, and usual activities. Patients report their level of difficulty in performing each task on a scale of 0 (without any difficulty), 1 (with some difficulty), 2 (with much difficulty), and 3 (unable to do). It can be modified to assess spondylitis-specific measures (HAQ-S). It has also been modified to assess the severity of psoriatic arthritis.

SpA-adjusted HAQ contains 5 additional items to the original HAQ in recognition of the functional importance of neck rotation.

BASMI (Bath AS Metrology Index) is a reproducible and sensitive method for assessing spinal mobility. It measures neck rotation and any forward stooping of the neck, lumbar spinal forward bending (using modified Schöber's test), and lateral bending of the lumbar spine (using fingertip-to-floor distance, and ability to spread legs maximally apart while lying down on the examining table. These scores also range from 0 to 10, and higher scores indicate greater impairment.

BASRI (Bath AS Radiology Index) is a system of scoring radiographic change, but it has been superseded by *mSASSS* (modified Stoke AS Spondylitis Spine Score) that evaluates the anterior vertebral edges of the neck and lumbar spine by grading the presence of chronic changes using a score ranging from 0 (no damage) to 3 (complete bony bridging/fusion between two adjacent vertebrae).

Health-Related Quality of Life (HR-QoL) measures

ASAS HI is a relatively new and preferred "all in one" index (clinical instrument) to keep track of changes in the overall health status of patients with AS/axSpA and other forms of SpA. It includes patients' responses about their pain, fatigue, and limitation in activities and social participation that are not adequately captured and assessed by other currently used questionnaires. ASDAS app is available free-of-charge on the Apple App Store and Google Play.

AS QoL (AS Quality of Life) is a patient-reported disease-specific 18-item questionnaire measuring pain, fatigue, function, and emotion in patients with AS. It is mostly being replaced by the better and free-of-charge ASAS HI.

SF-36 (Short-Study Form-36) is a self-administered questionnaire that has been widely used for many different diseases to measure physical and psychological dimensions of quality of life (QoL). It consists of 36 questions broken down into 8 physical and mental domains of quality of life: physical functioning, pain, role limitations due to physical problems, role limitations due to emotional problems, mental health, social functioning, energy/fatigue, and general health perceptions. Through a somewhat complicated system of scoring, the first 4 of these 8 domains give the physical component score (PCS) and the remaining 4 give the mental component score (MCS) of quality of life.

Mental Health (Depression): Depression is assessed with the Center for Epidemiological Studies Depression (CES-D) Scale, a 20-item questionnaire measuring depressive symptomatology over the preceding 1 week.

PASS (Patient-Acceptable Symptom State) is a reliable and valid tool for health assessment simply asking the patient the following question and requesting only a "yes" or "no" answer: "Considering all the different ways your disease is affecting you, if you would stay in this state for the next months, do you consider that your current state is satisfactory?"

WAPI (Work Productivity and Activity Impairment) questionnaire measures the impact of disease on the amount of work-related *absenteeism* (reflecting time away from scheduled work), *presenteeism* (reflecting reduced productivity while at work), *overall work impairment* (the sum of absenteeism and presenteeism), and *activity impairment* (reflecting ability to perform daily non-work-related activities).

WLQ-25 (Work Limitations Questionnaire-25) contains 25-item to assess 4 dimensions of presenteeism: physical demands (6 questions), time management demands (5 questions), mental-interpersonal demands (9 questions), and output demands (5 questions).

13

Patient education

 Key points

- For people living with AS/axSpA, a chronic illness for which there is as yet no cure, the future is filled with uncertainty.

- Patients deserve receiving the appropriate education and counseling about their illness from their doctor, and their concerns need to be addressed. The word "doctor" does not mean a healer but an educator.

- With the increasing use of electronic medical record (EMR) systems, many healthcare providers seem to be spending more time looking at their computer screens and clicking their keyboards rather than looking at and conversing with their patients during their clinic visits.

- Internet-empowered digital communications strategies have proven to be efficient in disseminating information on specific topics by medical associations, patient advocacy groups, and organizations.

- The patients should be as actively involved in their treatment process as possible and not simply be passive recipients of medical services, and they also need psychologic support through conversation that includes elements of empathy, honesty, and trust. This will strengthen the clinician-patient relationship.

Introduction

With the increasing use of electronic medical record (EMR) systems, many healthcare providers seem to be spending more time looking at their computer screens and clicking at their keyboards rather than looking at and conversing with their patients during their clinic visits. People living with AS/axSpA, a long-standing (chronic) illness for which there is as yet no cure and its precise cause not yet fully defined, face a future filled with uncertainty, made worse by

Ankylosing Spondylitis and Axial Spondyloarthritis, Second Edition. Muhammad Asim Khan, Oxford University Press.
© Oxford University Press 2023. DOI: 10.1093/oso/9780198864158.003.0013

accusations of laziness or imagined illness. It is imperative for the healthcare providers to know that humans enjoy being around someone who will listen to their problems attentively without casting judgement.

Patients need psychologic support through conversation that includes elements of empathy, honesty, and trust. That trust in your physician will increase and you will feel at ease if your concerns are listened to and addressed and you receive appropriate education and counseling about your illness. Patients who are better educated about their illness have better outcomes.

The word "doctor" implies an educator, not a healer. Thus, the Doctor of Philosophy (PhD) degree was originally granted to learned individuals who had achieved an approval of their peers by demonstrating a long and productive career in the field of philosophy (in the broad sense of the term, meaning the pursuit of knowledge). But in the English language the word "doctor" has long had a secondary meaning to indicate a physician. Your rheumatologists should provide you with the truth about your illness, its likely outcome, and any potential untoward effects of the prescribed treatments.

You should be actively involved in the treatment process and not simply be a passive recipients of medical services. The rheumatologist and the patient should form a team working toward the same goals: greater comfort, increased functionality, and improved quality of life. In a survey of 2,486 patients from 17 European countries living with AS/axSpA, approximately one-third had not talked to their clinician about their personal treatment goals.

The Internet

The "digital revolution" and the Internet age have led to modernization of the patient education and knowledge-diffusion process. These developments have resulted in younger generations seeking knowledge about their health-related issues from "Dr Google." This trend is fostered by the availability of many information sources and the changing role of healthcare professionals.

You should be selective and "not believe everything that washes ashore while you are surfing the Net." There is a lot of misinformation out there that can be harmful. As these new tools for the acquisition and spread of medical knowledge become better understood by physicians and patients, interest in their proper use will continue to increase. They will improve public health and provide access to appropriate medical information for patients.

Medicine has traditionally valued privacy, confidentiality, and one-on-one interaction, but social media fosters openness that seems to contradict the concept of medical professionalism. However, the strategic use of social media seems to have many benefits, such as keeping participants updated in a practical and dynamic manner through sharing and spreading of relevant information quickly and efficiently and providing a new way of communication with patients and improving their medical follow-up.

The emerging field of *Digital Health*, also called *TeleHealth* and *Mobile Health*, helps organize and improve health services via the Internet and related computer technologies, and also the sharing of appropriate information with patients to establish a new form of communication and follow-up, including "*virtual visits*" to healthcare providers. Health- and social-care professionals are now using a wide range of *virtual* communities for their continuing professional education and information sharing. These media have also encouraged patients to take on an essential role in their healthcare, and this has led to an important new concept called the "*E-patient*" where the first letter E can refer to an *equipped, enabled, engaged, empowered,* and *expert* patient.

The current deadly COVID-19 pandemic has further increased interest and participation by patients in Internet-empowered digital communication strategies that have proven to be quite efficient and effective in disseminating information on specific topics by healthcare providers, patient advocacy groups, medical associations, and other organizations.

14

Exercise and physical therapy

 Key points

- There are non-pharmacological modalities in the form of physical exercises (unsupervised or supervised single or group physical exercises (on ground and/or in water)) that complement the current availability of remarkably effective pharmacological therapies.

- Life-long regular physical exercise regimen and proper posture control are generally underutilized by patients as well as their healthcare providers, although they are of fundamental importance in the successful long-term management of AS/axSpA and preventing or minimizing spinal stiffness and deformity.

- Randomized controlled trials have shown that physiotherapy with disease education is effective in the treatment of people with AS/axSpA, and group physical therapy is cost-effective compared to individualized therapy.

- Patients' posture problems and difficulties in performing activities of daily living should be identified, and workplace modifications may be needed.

- Self-help programs and patient education and counseling improve patients' compliance with therapy regimens and benefit their general health and functional status. At minimum, any physical activity is better than no activity. You should avoid any neck or back manipulation by a chiropractor or a massage therapist. Use of back splints, braces, and corsets is not helpful and should be avoided.

Ankylosing Spondylitis and Axial Spondyloarthritis, Second Edition. Muhammad Asim Khan, Oxford University Press.
© Oxford University Press 2023. DOI: 10.1093/oso/9780198864158.003.0014

Introduction

Regular physical exercises are of fundamental importance in the successful long-term management of AS/axSpA. They aim to maintain or to improve correct posture and mobility of the neck, back, hip, and shoulder; prevent and decrease tightening (shortening) of muscle and ligaments; and minimize deformity. They also ease pain, improve physical functioning, lung capacity, chest expansion, health status, and quality of life.

Physicians should educate patients about the role of such exercises and provide them with written instructions or pamphlets with illustrations about proper posture maintenance and appropriate home-based exercises that are easy to perform and are convenient and free. This is facilitated by arranging an initial formal physiotherapy consultation, especially as a source of information about proper posture, appropriate exercises, and recreational sports, and the need for maintaining a regular life-long exercise program.

The physiotherapist can suggest and teach you the physical exercises and recreational sports that are best for you, and you should strive to do them routinely. Try to do at least some of the exercises every day. Because the disease severity and course are different among patients, therapeutic exercises must be tailored to your degree of spinal mobility or involvement.

Most patients feel too stiff to exercise in the morning, although taking a warm bath before exercising tends to ease this discomfort. Choose a time of the day that works best for you. A warm shower before exercising also tends to promote relaxation and helps in passive stretching of tight muscles. If you have pain during or after your exercises, consult your rheumatologist. With determination, regular exercises, sometimes combined with a program of stretching and muscle strengthening, will make you feel fitter and retain good range of movement of spine, hip, and shoulder joints. Gentle stretching exercises ease stiffness and help prevent postural changes, and muscle-strengthening exercises help in retaining proper posture. Passive stretching of the hip joints increases their range of movement and thus improves function and posture.

Physical exercises complement the current availability of remarkably effective pharmacological therapy, but these non-pharmacological modalities are generally under-utilized by patients and physicians. Cigarette smoking should be strongly discouraged because it is associated with worse outcomes. Self-help programs and patient education and counseling improve patients' compliance with therapy regimens and benefit their general health and functional status.

People who comply with a comprehensive medical management program that includes a lifetime of daily exercises can help maintain satisfactory spinal mobility. However, even with optimal treatment, some people will develop a stiff spine, but they will remain functional even if the spine fuses in an upright position, as long as they have minimal impairment of mobility of their limb joints.

A yearly follow-up visit to a physiotherapist can ensure that these exercises are being performed appropriately; this can also keep track of any improvement or worsening in physical posture and joint and spine range of motion. Back stretching and deep breathing exercises, swimming and water aerobics, stationary bicycling, and other appropriate recreational exercises are especially useful. They can help enhance general fitness, lung capacity, exercise capability, muscle strength, and range of motion. They also increase cardiovascular conditioning and endurance. Patients with heart disease should be assessed by their physician and may require an exercise tolerance test before starting to exercise. You should avoid any neck or back manipulation by a chiropractor or a massage therapist.

Patients' posture problems and difficulties in performing activities of daily living should be identified, and workplace modifications may be needed. Frequently changing position when sitting at a desk and taking breaks for body stretching are helpful. Activities that cause back muscle strain should be avoided (e.g., prolonged stooping or bending and assuming positions that may cause a stooped posture, such as prolonged slouching in chairs or leaning over a desk).

Helpful assistive devices include long-handled devices for dressing and for reaching for objects or picking items from the floor or very low places by using "grabbers". Adjustable swivel chairs that provide lumbar support, and adjustable writing or working desk surfaces may also be needed (Figure 20.2). Use of wide-view mirrors can be helpful for patients with limited neck mobility when driving (see Chapter 21 for further discussions). Use of back splints, braces, and corsets is not helpful and should be avoided.

Swimming

Swimming is an ideal exercise for those who enjoy it because it gently uses all the muscles and is very relaxing. It provides aerobic exercise to enhance general fitness and improve lung capacity. A warm or even hot pool is generally most comfortable. A heated swimming pool or spa helps to decrease pain and stiffness and therefore allows you to perform exercises when it might otherwise be impossible because of the pain. Low-impact exercises (swimming and water aerobics) and stationary bicycling can help improve exercise capability, muscle strength, and range of motion. You should be very careful not to slip on wet surfaces in the pool area, and it is also wise to avoid diving into the pool. Patients with active psoriasis should avoid chlorinated water.

Regular freestyle swimming is considered to be one of the best exercises for people with AS, but if your neck is rigid, it may be difficult to swim freestyle. Using a snorkel may be helpful, provided you swim only under observation and near the edge of a swimming pool if it is deep. This precaution is necessary because someone with limited breathing capacity may not be able to blow the water out effectively if it inadvertently enters the snorkel tube. In some European countries, professionally supervised special physiotherapy group sessions organized by AS patient societies and group exercise sessions at a spa or hydrotherapy center are enjoyable and very helpful. Randomized controlled trials have shown that physiotherapy with disease education is effective in the treatment of people with AS, and group physical therapy is cost-effective compared to individualized therapy.

Application of heat

A warm shower or application of local heat may promote relaxation and help in passive stretching of tight muscles. You should not apply local heat to an area for more than 15 minutes at a time. Avoid areas overlying artificial joints. Keep the temperature setting of the heating pad at low or medium level, never on high setting. Do not lie on a heating pad to apply heat to your back to avoid skin burn that can result, in part, from decreased blood circulation in the area due to pressure of your body weight.

Spinal extension and deep breathing exercises

A general set of routine exercises to be performed at home is discussed here, and a physiotherapist can advise you of the exercises that are most suitable for you, based on the severity of your diseases and resultant physical limitations. The aim to prevent or decrease incorrect posture, improve strength, and avoid contractures (shortening) of muscles, and improve mobility of spine, hip and shoulder joints.

You can start by performing spinal extension combined with breathing exercises from a lying position with face down (lying on your front), with your arms stretched by your side. Then, while drawing your shoulder blades together, raise your head, chest, shoulders, and arms off the bed as far as possible while taking a deep breath in (Figure 14.1). Hold your body in that position for about 5 seconds and then relax and breath out. You may put a pillow under your chest but not your belly, to make it easier to perform this exercise. Repeat the exercise about 10 times.

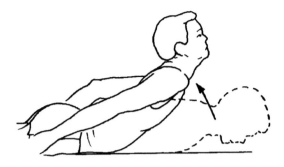

Figure 14.1 Extension of the neck and back from lying position.

While lying down face down on your front, you can also turn your head to one side, arms by your side, raise one leg off the ground while keeping the knee straight and trying to raise your thigh off the ground (figure not shown). Repeat on each leg 5 times.

You can also perform the chest expansion and deep breathing exercise while standing erect with knees straight and feet wide apart (Figure 14.2a), preferably with your back against a wall, and back of the heel touching the wall. It can also be performed while lying on your back (Figure 14.2b). First raise the arms sideways and then all the way up and your elbows fully extended, while taking a deep breath in. Hold the breath for a count of 10 before exhaling and relaxing for about 10 seconds. Repeat the exercise about 10 times. If you are a smoker, you need to give up smoking in order to prevent its adverse effects on the lungs and heart.

You can combine spinal extension and stretching with chest wall expansion by performing corner push-ups (Figure 14.3), in which you face a corner and place your hands on the opposing walls at shoulder height. Then bend your elbows to lean forward towards the corner with your head, neck, and spine fully extended, knees fully stretched, and heels touching the ground. Take in a deep breath during this maneuver and hold your breath for a count of 10. Then exhale while returning to the upright position. Repeat this exercise about 20 times, up to 3 times daily if possible.

Muscle-strengthening and stretching exercises

Exercises to strengthen the extensor muscles of the back and hip can be performed in water or on land. You should try to achieve a functional range of motion of the hip and shoulder joints. Severe loss of motion of hip joints can

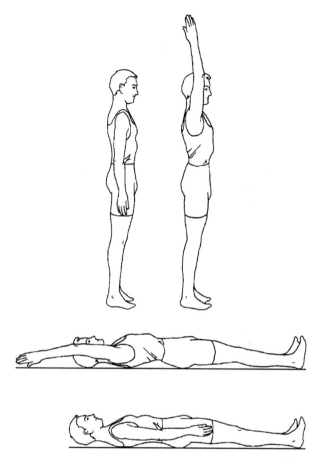

Figure 14.2 Deep breathing exercises while standing and when lying on the back.

be more disabling than a fused spine. Specific exercises such as daily stretching of involved joints may be needed to improve mobility of the back, hips, shoulders, or other involved joints. Physical exercises are needed to keep your joints from getting stiff, to regain muscle strength, and prevent muscle wasting and weakness.

Detailed discussion about maintaining proper posture are provided in Chapter 21. You should sleep on your back on a firm bed with a thin pillow under your neck (and head). In the morning and at the end of each day, you should lie on

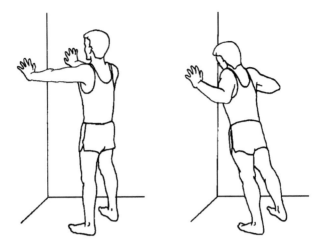

Figure 14.3 Corner push-ups for anterior chest wall expansion and deep breathing as well as stretching of the back.

Reprinted with kind permission from *Straight Talk on Spondylitis*, published by the Spondylitis Association of America.

your front (face down) for up to 15 minutes, if possible, in order to prevent contracture (bending) at your hips and knees. Another way to stretch your back and hip joints is to lie on your back at the side of the bed with your legs dangling to the floor.

This next exercise, shown as Figure 14.4, can be called "bridge making," and is performed to stretch and strengthen the hip region. Do not perform this exercise if it causes neck pain while doing it. First lie down on your back and bend both knees and place your feet flat on the floor. Then maximally lift your hip off the floor, hold for 5 seconds, and then slowly lower your hips down.

Figure 14.5 illustrates back stretching and mobility exercise on all four limbs ("cat back and sway"). Kneel on all fours, keeping the forearms straight, and then hump up your back as high as you can, with the head bent down. Then arch your back and raise your head as much as you can for a slow count of 5. Then stretch alternate arms and legs parallel to the floor and hold for a slow count of 10. Then lower and repeat this exercise using the other limbs.

The following exercises are performed while sitting on a chair without armrests. Figure 14.6 shows chest and back lateral flexion, body rotation, and neck rotation to the right side. These are then repeated on the left side (figures not shown). This is followed by forward bending (flexion) of the neck (figure not shown) by trying to bring the chin closest to the front of the chest, and then

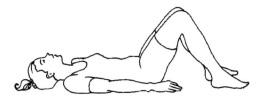

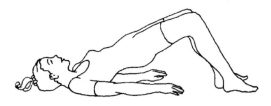

Figure 14.4 Bridge-making exercise.

Reproduced with permission from "A positive response to ankylosing Spondylitis—A guidebook for patients", produced by the Royal National Hospital for Rheumatic Diseases, Bath, 1998.

try to look upwards (extension). Figure 14.7 demonstrates exercises to stretch the hamstring (muscles in the back of the leg) and the quadriceps (the thigh muscles) in the legs.

Sports and recreational activities

Sports and recreational activities that encourage good posture as well as encourage arching of the back (extension) and rotation of the trunk are recommended (please read Chapter 21 for additional discussions). These include walking, hiking, swimming, tennis, badminton, cross-country skiing, and archery. If you have neck involvement you need to be more careful and follow safety instructions. High-impact and contact sports activities and those that involve abrupt movement of the spine should be avoided, especially by patients who have limited spinal mobility. Sports activities that require prolonged spinal flexion, including golfing, bowling, and long-distance cycling, may be inadvisable.

Body contact sports (such as boxing, rugby, hockey, soccer, and American football) and downhill skiing are not recommended because of their greater potential for injury. Stationary bike exercises are good but the handlebars

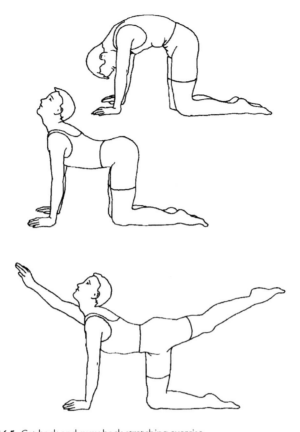

Figure 14.5 Cat back and sway back stretching exercise.

Reproduced with permission from "A positive response to ankylosing Spondylitis—a guidebook for patients", produced by the Royal National Hospital for Rheumatic Diseases, Bath, 1998.

must be properly adjusted so that you do not lean forward while exercising. This exercise is especially good for general cardiovascular conditioning, strengthening the leg muscles, and exercising the hip and knee joints. Aerobic exercises with machines that enhance back, leg, and shoulder extension are helpful, but you should avoid undue stress on the neck. Volleyball and basketball (with a little lower net or basket and specially adapted rules) are excellent sports for people with AS because they combine movement with stretching (Figure 14.8). However, not everyone can tolerate jarring activities.

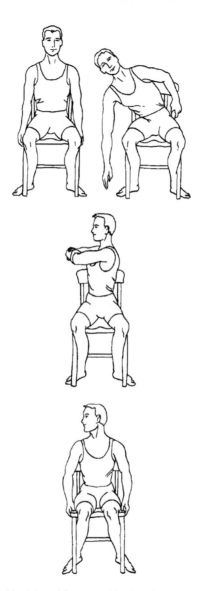

Figure 14.6 Chest and back lateral flexion, and body and neck rotation to the right side.
Reproduced with permission from "A positive response to ankylosing Spondylitis—A guidebook for patients", produced by the Royal National Hospital for Rheumatic Diseases, Bath, 1998.

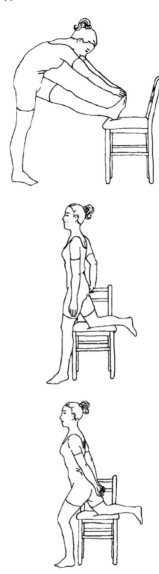

Figure 14.7 Exercises to stretch the hamstring and quadricep muscles.
Reproduced with permission from "A positive response to ankylosing Spondylitis—A guidebook for patients", produced by the Royal National Hospital for Rheumatic Diseases, Bath, 1998.

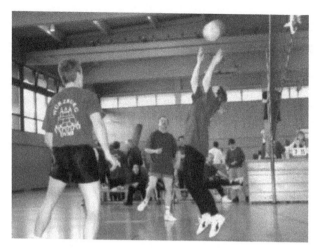

Figure 14.8 Volleyball with specially adapted rules as practiced in local groups of AS organizations (here of the German AS society) is an excellent sport for people with AS because it combines movement with stretching.

Reproduced from *Bechterew-Brief*, the newsletter of DVMB, No. 78 (September 1999), p. 15. © Deutsche Vereinigung Morbus Bechterew, Schweinfurt.

Mind-body relaxation exercises

Tai Chi is a traditional Chinese mind–body relaxation exercise consisting of 108 intricate exercise sequences performed in a slow relaxed manner over a 30-minute period. A study from China has shown that, compared with the standard exercise therapy, "Tai Chi spinal exercise therapy" more effectively relieves low back pain and improves the back muscle function and balance in patients with AS.

Yoga is an Indian spiritual discipline that includes simple meditation, awareness, and control over respiration (breathing), and specific body (psycho-physical) postures intended to create harmony between mind, body and environment. It is commonly considered to be an exercise system for general fitness and well-being. Its proponents claim that regular yoga exercises can help maintain spinal and general flexibility and mobility, and also lower stress and ease pain, thus resulting in an improved quality of life for those with AS and related forms of SpA.

Barriers to performing regular exercises

The main reasons may be the general lack of motivation on the part of the patients and the lack of appropriate centers for physical exercises and recreation. Some patients notice worsening of pain when they exercise, or they may not be convinced about the benefits of exercise. Others may fear that the exercise may worsen their disease, or face barriers such as safety concerns, lack of social support, finances, or time. Lastly, the healthcare providers may not be conveying to their patients the very beneficial effects of physical exercises.

15

Management

An overview

 Key points

- There is currently no preventive measure or a curative treatment for AS/axSpA, but in most people the disease can be very well managed.

- Early diagnosis and effective therapeutic interventions markedly improve the outcome.

- All patients should be provided with disease-specific written instructions and illustrations in the form of handouts, books, or pamphlets, or as videos, audiotapes, and information about useful websites.

- Regular range of motion exercise is of fundamental importance in preventing or minimizing stiffness and deformity.

- There are many AS self-help and support groups that enlist enthusiastic patient cooperation, provide information about the disease and advice about life and health insurance, jobs, working environment, and other useful items.

- Patients are advised to carry a "medical alert" or "personal information" card that contains concise important information about them.

Introduction

There is currently no preventive measure or a curative treatment for AS/axSpA, but in most people the disease can be very well managed. Early and more precise diagnosis leads to earlier and more rational or effective therapeutic interventions. The severity of disease symptoms and the degree of joint involvement vary greatly from one person to another. Several drugs are used in treating AS/

Ankylosing Spondylitis and Axial Spondyloarthritis, Second Edition. Muhammad Asim Khan, Oxford University Press.
© Oxford University Press 2023. DOI: 10.1093/oso/9780198864158.003.0015

axSpA. They do not cure the disease but most help in minimizing pain and maintaining mobility and function. The information about drug therapy provided in this and the next 5 chapters is only a guideline. You should ask your doctor and pharmacist about the dose and how and when to take any prescribed drugs, and also inquire about their potential untoward effects.

Cessation of cigarette smoking should be strongly advised because smoking is associated with impaired response to treatment and worse outcomes. Patients who are markedly overweight or obese need weight reduction because they also carry worst outcomes and poor response to treatment.

Regular range of motion exercise is of fundamental importance in preventing or minimizing stiffness and deformity. Spinal extension and deep breathing exercises should be done routinely once or twice daily. People with AS should walk erect, keeping the spine as straight as possible, and sleep on a firm mattress using a thin pillow, just thick enough to allow a horizontal position of the face to prevent pain from overextension of the neck. Physical activity that places prolonged strain on back muscles, such as prolonged bending and stooping, or prolonged slouching in chairs, or leaning over a desk should be avoided. Frequently changing position when sitting at a desk and taking breaks for body stretching are helpful. Adjustable swivel chairs that provide lumbar support, and elevated and inclined writing surfaces are very helpful.

People with limited spinal mobility should avoid physical-contact sports and physical trauma or falls because even a trivial injury can result in fracture. Manipulation of their back or neck by chiropractors or masseurs should also be avoided because it can inadvertently result in spinal fractures. Use of back splints, braces, and corsets is not helpful and should be avoided. Those with posture problems and difficulties in performing activities of daily living should be identified, and workplace modifications may be needed.

Formal physiotherapy is of value for learning the proper physical posture, appropriate exercises and recreational sports, and the importance of maintaining a regular exercise program. All patients should be provided with disease-specific written instructions about proper posture and appropriate home-based exercises and encouraged to perform them regularly. Group exercise sessions that include warm water exercises (hydrotherapy) are very helpful. If they can, water-based exercises are to be recommended because swimming (especially freestyle or back stroke) is one of the best exercises.

There are many *AS/axSpA self-help groups or organizations* that provide illustrated handouts, books and pamphlets, or videos, patient education, and counseling to improve patients' compliance with therapy regimens and improve their general health and well-being as well their functional status. Some of them can also provide advice about life and health insurance, jobs, and working environment (see Appendix 1 for contact details). They also provide information about some helpful assistive devices that include wide-view mirrors (for car driving), long-handled devices for reaching or picking objects, or for assistance in dressing.

Total hip joint replacement (THR), also called total hip arthroplasty (THA), gives very good results and prevents partial or total disability from severe hip disease (see Chapter 23, Figure 23.1). Heart complications may require pacemaker implantation and/or aortic valve replacement (see Chapter 7). Vertebral wedge bone resection may be needed to correct the severe stooping deformity that may occasionally occur, although this surgery carries a relatively high risk of paralysis of legs (paraplegia).

Patients should also be advised to keep their *vaccination status* up to date and receive yearly influenza vaccinations, as well as proper vaccination against

Medical Alert Card for Patients With AS *(especially those with advanced disease)*			CAUTION: My whole spine is fused (rigid), including my neck. I am prone to easily fracturing my neck or my back, and it can happen even after a trivial injury. Spinal fracture, if it is unstable or is not properly immobilized, *can lead to paralysis or death.*
My Name & Contact Information	I suffer from ankkylosing spondylitits, a form of arthritis that has caused a sever limitation of motion of my back and neck.	NAME	Be careful to avoid any movement of my neck and back while lifting me onto a stretcher or an examining table, and during any procedure, such as radiography (x-rays) or insertion of a tube in the windpipe (trachea) for breathing or general anesthesia. My rib cage is also fused, therefore I have very limited chest expansion. I breathe mainly by using my diaphragm.
	My home and/or work phone, including area code are:	HOME	
		WORK	
ICE & Medical Contacts	In case of emergency (ICE), call:	NAME	Before any x-ray or other imaging studies (MR or CT), my fused (rigid) and forwardly stooped neck or any part of my spine **MUST** be kept in its usual alignment (during conventional immobilization by emergency services before radiographic or surgical procedures).
		PHONE	
	My physician/hospital information:	NAME	
		PHONE	
		FAX	
		e-MAIL	

Allergies/Medications /Illnesses	I am allergic to:		My neck is forwardly stooped by roughly _____ degrees.
	My dailiy medications include:		CAUTION: Excessive straightening of my neck or spine into a "normal" position can make a stable fracture unstable and *may result in paralysis or death.* Plain x-rays of the neck and the back may not detect the fracture, and it may require MRI or CT.
	My other illnesses (besides AS) include:		

For additional information on my disease, suitable websites include:
www.spondylitis.org, www.spondyloarthritis-international.org, and www.bechterew.ch

Figure 15.1 Examples of a medical alert card for patients with AS/axSpA

COVID-19, including booster doses of the vaccine as needed, because properly vaccinated individuals are 8 times less likely to get the disease and 25 times less likely to require hospitalization or die from the disease. It is reassuring to know that AS/axSpA *per se* does not appear to confer a higher susceptibility to COVID-19. The US Center for Disease Control and Prevention (CDC) has advised that "people with immunocompromising conditions or people who take immunosuppressive medications or therapies are at increased risk for severe COVID-19. Because the immune response following COVID-19 vaccination may differ in people who are moderately or severely immunocompromised at the time of vaccination", specific guidance is available at <https://www.cdc.gov/vaccines/covid-19/clinical-considerations/interim-considerations-us.html#immunocompromised>.

Medical Alert Card: Patients are advised to carry a "medical alert" or "personal information" card (see Chapter 22) that contains concise information about them, including their emergency contact, medications, list of allergies, health insurance information, and blood type. My proposed version is shown in Figure 15.1 that can be adapted and will be of use to healthcare providers in case of an emergency situation.

16

Management

Patient's role

 Key points

- The long-term outcome is better for the patients whose disease gets diagnosed at an early stage and are managed by rheumatologists.

- Every newly diagnosed patient should be educated about the disease they have, and how to treat it. Depression and anxiety are not uncommon among patients, and these are treatable diseases that have many underlying causes. Some individuals are genetically prone to depression.

- Beyond prescribed medicine, there is an aspect called self-management that aims to provide the patient and their families with the support they need in order to achieve and maintain physical independence.

- You should feel free to discuss any issues related not only to your job and employment but also your personal life (such as sexual life, self-image, marriage, reproductive health, fertility, and pregnancy).

- It is important for you to tell your healthcare providers about any herbs, "over-the counter" medicines (not needing any prescriptions), megavitamins, prebiotics, probiotics, and any potentially addictive substances that you may be using.

- Co-management of your disease involves working with your rheumatologist, primary care physician, and appropriate specialists for any associated manifestations (such as uveitis, IBD, and psoriasis) or comorbid conditions (such as hypertension, obesity, and diabetes).

Ankylosing Spondylitis and Axial Spondyloarthritis, Second Edition. Muhammad Asim Khan, Oxford University Press.
© Oxford University Press 2023. DOI: 10.1093/oso/9780198864158.003.0016

Introduction

Every newly diagnosed patient should be made aware about the disease they have and how to treat it, but an important aspect of living with AS/axSpA, beyond the prescribed medicine, is your ability to manage daily physical, cultural, and emotional consequences of the illness, and any changes in lifestyle and employment. This is called self-management and it aims to provide you the support you need to achieve and maintain independence. You should know the primary goal of best management of AS/axSpA is to maximize the long-term, health-related quality of life through 3 objectives:

◆ Controlling symptoms and inflammation

◆ Preventing progressive structural damage

◆ Preserving or normalizing function and social participation

Optimal management mandates a combination of non-pharmacologic and pharmacologic treatment clearly explained to you (and your family) in printed and/or online form so that you gain knowledge about your illness. This will enhance your compliance with the recommended treatment, which is essential for the best outcome. You should discuss the efficacy and the impact of the various treatment options and their expected outcome and inquire about the impact of the disease on your family members. It is not unusual for more than one person in a family to be affected by AS or related diseases, so tell the physician in detail about the family history in case the physician forgets to ask you about it. You may want to know about the odds that your children may also develop the disease.

The long-term outcome is better for patients whose disease gets diagnosed at an early stage and they are managed by rheumatologists, with monitoring of disease activity and any adverse effects of drug therapies. The best management strategy used by rheumatologists incorporates individualized treatment and use of medications based on your current disease manifestations, the level of your current symptoms, clinical findings, disease activity and severity, functional status, deformities, general health status, comorbid conditions, disease-coping strategies, and your wishes and expectations.

You should keep a list of all the medicine you take, and also a list of drugs that you are allergic or intolerant to. It is important for you to share with your healthcare providers any "over-the-counter" (OTC) medicines (not needing any prescription), herbal supplements, megavitamins, probiotics, prebiotics, and potentially addictive substances that you may be using. Probiotics and prebiotics are discussed in Chapter 23.

A recent survey of a very large number of patients reaffirms the need to incorporate the patient's perspective to facilitate shared decision-making between patients and physicians. This results in better physical and psychological health outcomes due to improved patient participation in their own care and greater adherence with the prescribed treatment.

A life-long program of regular physical exercise, including home-based exercises that can be easily performed and are convenient and cost-free, is vital. Referral to a physical therapist is needed for specific instructions for spinal extension, deep breathing, and range of motion exercises of the back, neck, hips, and shoulders and other joints. A yearly follow-up visit with the physical therapist can ensure that the physical exercises are being performed accurately; and this can also help track any worsening of physical posture and mobility. Lifestyle and workplace modifications may also be needed.

Co-management of your disease with your primary care physician and appropriate specialists for any associated uveitis, psoriasis, IBD or comorbid conditions (hypertension, obesity, diabetes) is important. In cases of acute anterior uveitis, consultation with an ophthalmologist is urgently needed. Some patients have inadequate sleep due to worsened back pain and stiffness at night, or from obstructive sleep apnea that may require use of BIPAP/CPAP machines at night. Orthopedic consultation may be needed for elective THA in patients with advanced hip joint involvement causing severe pain or functional disability, and emergency consultation may be needed after physical injury and suspected spinal fracture.

I have mentioned many times in this book that it is important for you to quit tobacco use (smoking) because it worsens your disease outcome as well as its adverse effect on heart and lungs.

You should feel free to discuss any issues related not only to your job and employment but also your personal life (such as sexual life, self-image, marriage, reproductive health, fertility, and pregnancy). Depression and anxiety as well as fibromyalgia are not uncommon among patients with any chronic painful illness that impairs quality of life. It is important for you to know that depression is a potentially treatable disease that has many underlying causes, and that some individuals are genetically prone to depression.

17

Management

Rheumatologist's role

 Key points

- Rheumatologists are board-certified internists with an additional two or 3 years of fellowship training to diagnose and treat arthritis and other musculoskeletal diseases.

- Their most important role is not only to diagnose an illness and prescribe appropriate treatment, but also to monitor and adjust such therapy when appropriate and educate and provide counselling to patients and their families.

- Well-established rheumatology centers have physician assistants, nurse practitioners, specialist nurses, physiotherapists, occupational therapists, and medical social workers.

- They may also work closely with other health professionals such as physiatrists, orthopedists, podiatrists, psychiatrists, psychologists, pharmacists, and dieticians.

- It is important for you to be made aware that your perspective will be incorporated by your rheumatologist for "shared decision-making", and this also involves your primary care physician or internist.

Introduction

Rheumatologists are physicians uniquely educated and trained to diagnose and treat arthritis and other diseases of the joints, muscles, and bones. In the US, a rheumatologist is a board-certified internist (internal medicine specialist) or a board-certified pediatrician who has had an additional 2–3 years of specialized rheumatology training. These physicians can then become "board-certified" in rheumatology after passing another board certification examination. They are therefore highly trained specialists in diagnosing and treating arthritis and other rheumatic diseases.

Rheumatologists based in academic centers or hospital-based rheumatology units help to train other doctors and allied health professionals in addition to providing care to their own patients. They are often also involved in conducting clinical and basic scientific research in rheumatic diseases. Most rheumatologists, however, are in private practice, although some of them have clinical affiliations with academic medical centers and also conduct clinical research and/or drug trials.

The well-established rheumatology units or centers include not only rheumatologists but also trained allied health professionals such as physician assistants, nurse practitioners, specialist nurses, physiotherapists, occupational therapists, and medical social workers. They also work closely with other health professionals such as orthopedists, physiatrists, podiatrists, psychiatrists, psychologists, pharmacists, and dieticians.

In an ideal setting, a patient sees his/her PCP, GP, internists, or another healthcare provider who performs baseline clinical screening (history, physical examination, and testing). The patient is referred to a rheumatologist if AS/axSpA is suspected to ensure proper diagnosis and management. Ideally, the patient should then be examined by a rheumatologist within 3 weeks of the referral but it is often not possible because of a shortage of rheumatologists in most countries.

The rheumatologist's most important role is to decide on the diagnosis and explain the illness to the patient, its long-term impact, especially if left untreated, and an appropriate treatment plan. For those reasons, a rheumatologist will ask about detailed medical history, including family history, social history (such as occupation, hobbies, travels, smoking, and use of illicit drugs), and history of other illnesses or surgeries before carrying out a clinical examination. Afterwards, blood tests and X-rays (or other forms of imaging, such as MRI) may need to be ordered to arrive at a decide and how best to treat the patient.

It is wise to get the relevant medical notes and a letter of referral from your PCP/internist and also bring with you, if you can, your previous medical records and any imaging results. Also bring a list of the medication that you are currently taking or have previously taken, a list of your vaccinations, and your drug allergy history. Do not hesitate to bring someone with you to the rheumatologist's office, if you prefer, especially during your first visit. Do not hesitate to ask any questions you may have.

Patient's concerns and shared decision-making

What matters most to patients is their pain, limitation of physical function, fatigue, feeling of exhaustion, impaired sleep, decreased motivation, difficulty in walking or standing for long, concerns about their emotional well-being and social interactions, and potential side effects of prescribed treatment.

It is important for you to be made aware that your perspective will be incorporated by your rheumatologist for "shared decision-making", and this also involves your PCP. You should be an active partner with your healthcare team as this can result in better physical and psychological health outcomes due to greater adherence with the prescribed treatment that includes a regular exercise program. Consistency rather than quantity of exercise is of utmost importance. It is the doctor's job to relieve your pain and stiffness, and your job to perform regular exercises and maintain a reasonably good posture. You can ask for any pamphlets, leaflets, or other information to help you gain better insight into your disease. You should also receive advice to help you to adopt a healthy lifestyle. If you are unhappy with or have doubts about your treatment, it is quite appropriate to ask for a second opinion from another consultant.

You should see your rheumatologist for periodic follow-up appointments, ideally at least every 3 to 6 months, at least for initial few visits. This is necessary to monitor disease activity and assess treatment response that may require guideline-based treatment adjustments. There should also be an annual comprehensive assessment. Many patients with AS/axSpA may need to be seen by their rheumatologist more frequently and over an extended period, rather than being cared for only by their PCP.

18

NSAIDs and
conventional DMARDs

 Key points

- NSAIDs are most often used to reduce pain and suppress inflammation as the first line of treatment for patients with AS/axSpA. They are not habit-forming, unlike narcotic pain relievers.

- The choice of the NSAIDs should be based on consideration of the patient's prior tolerance, risk factors for adverse effects on stomach, liver, or kidneys, and coexisting illnesses, such as high blood pressure and heart or kidney disease.

- Some of NSAIDs are available without a doctor's prescription ("over-the-counter") but at a lower strength (dose) than those available with a prescription.

- There is an increased risk of gastrointestinal bleeding from ulcers, especially among people over the age of 60, or with a previous history of peptic ulcer disease.

- Women who are pregnant or are breastfeeding should not take them without their doctor's advice.

- Conventional DMARDs are also called slow-acting anti-rheumatic drugs (SAARDs) because any benefit from these drugs takes some time to manifest. They include drugs such as sulfasalazine and methotrexate.

Introduction

Non-steroidal anti-inflammatory drugs (NSAIDs), other than acetyl salicylic acid (aspirin) and related salicylate compounds, are most often used to reduce

Ankylosing Spondylitis and Axial Spondyloarthritis, Second Edition. Muhammad Asim Khan, Oxford University Press.
© Oxford University Press 2023. DOI: 10.1093/oso/9780198864158.003.0018

pain and suppress inflammation as the first line of treatment for patients with symptomatic AS/axSpA. Patients seem to respond best if treated early in the course of disease, and they continue taking the medicine at the recommended dose. Their efficacy has been documented in multiple clinical trials in relieving back and limb joint pain and stiffness, and they also improve physical function. Moreover, they are not habit-forming, unlike narcotic pain relievers.

Approximately 50–80% of patients showed beneficial response from a study of 1,080 patients. The patients usually start noticing response within 1 to 2 weeks, but the drug that best controls the inflammation and pain may not be the first one that your doctor tries; a trial period may be needed to find the most effective NSAID for you. NSAIDs alone may not totally relieve pain and stiffness but provide enough relief at night that you should be able to get more restful sleep.

There are minimal differences in efficacy between the various NSAIDs, but there are some variations in their side effect profiles and drug interactions. The choice should be based on consideration of the patient's history of NSAID use, risk factors for adverse effects on stomach, liver, or kidneys, and comorbidities like high blood pressure and heart disease. The desirable effects far outweigh undesirable consequences for most, especially young patients. However, some patients are intolerant of or have contraindications to treatment with NSAIDs.

You should only take one NSAID at a time, in an adequate dose; using 2 or more NSAID at the same time increases the risk of side-effects without providing any additive benefit. If there is no response after 2 weeks or if you are intolerant, your physician may try another NSAID for another 2 weeks before discussing switching you to or adding biologic drugs, such as TNF inhibitors, to improve management of your disease. Tylenol and opioids do not control inflammation and therefore should not replace NSAIDs. Moreover, opioids are habit-forming (addictive), unlike the NSAIDs.

Not all the NSAIDs may be officially approved by the drug-regulating agencies for use in AS/axSpA in the various countries. Table 18.1 provides a list, in an alphabetic order, of most of the NSAIDs available in the US, with their generic names and some of their popular brand names that vary in different parts of the world. The brand name starts with a capital letter, but the generic (chemical) name does not. Several brand-name drugs can have the same generic name if they contain the same active ingredient. Thus, Motrin®, Advil®, Nuprin®, and Brufen® are the brand names for ibuprofen, whereas Aleve® and Anaprox® are the brand names for naproxen. These are available "over the counter" (without a doctor's prescription) in the US (but in lower strength) to relieve minor aches and pains. People with AS and related diseases need to take higher doses under a doctor's supervision. The longer-acting NSAIDs need to be taken only once or twice daily to enhance the patient's compliance. Do not take more than the prescribed dose.

Table 18.1 An incomplete list of NSAIDs approved in the US and some of them (such as ibuprofen and naproxen) are available in the US "over the counter," i.e., without a prescription. The brand names vary around the world, and those listed in parenthesis, such as Dolobid, are currently unavailable in the US.

Generic name	Brand name
Celecoxib	Celebrex
Diclofenac	Voltaren, Cataflam, Cambia
Diclofenac sodium plus misoprostol	Arthrotec
Diflunisal	(Dolobid)
Etodolac	(Lodine)
Fenoprofen Flurbiprofen	Nalfon Ansaid
Ibuprofen	Advil, Motrin, Nuprin
Indomethacin	Indocid, Indocin
Ketoprofen	(Orudis)
Ketorolac tromethamine	(Toradol)
Meclofenamate Mefenamic acid Meloxicam	Meclomen Ponstel Mobic
Nabumetone	(Relafen)
Naproxen	Aleve, Naprosyn, Naprelan
Naproxen sodium	Anaprox
Nimesulide Oxaprozin	(Sulide, Mesulid) Daypro
Piroxicam	Feldene
Tenoxicam Taprofenic acid Tolmetin	(Mobiflex) (Surgam) (Tolectin)
Sulindac	(Clinoril)

Side effects (untoward effects)

NSaids are relatively safe drugs but not all are equally tolerated, and responses as well as their untoward effects may differ. Therefore, you should inquire about the potential untoward effects (side effects) of NSAIDs from your doctor before their use. Women who are pregnant or are breastfeeding should not take them without their doctor's advice.

NSaids may interact with some other drugs, such as the blood thinner (anticoagulant) drug called warfarin (Coumadin®) and some other drugs such as methotrexate and lithium. Some of the NSAIDs may impair the function of blood cells called platelets, thereby increasing your susceptibility to bruising or prolonged bleeding from cuts or surgery. They can also cause fluid retention (most commonly manifested by swelling of the ankles), increase in blood pressure, or some blunting of the effect of drugs used to treat high blood pressure. On rare occasions there may be adverse effects on kidney or liver function, and a decrease in white or red blood cell count or other signs of bone marrow suppression.

Phenylbutazone (Butazolidin®) was one of the first and very effective NSAIDs but it is not used these days because of a potentially greater risk of bone marrow toxicity than the recent NSAIDs. Rofecoxib (Vioxx®) was also a very popular and effective drug, but it was withdrawn by its manufacturer from the US market because the FDA demanded additional safety data. Etoricoxib (Arcoxia®) and valdecoxib (Bextra®) were also withdrawn for similar reasons. However, rofecoxib and etoricoxib are still available in many countries, and the FDA gave rofecoxib an "orphan drug" designation in 2017 for the treatment of hemophilia associated arthritis for whom use of high-potency opioids had been the standard care in treating their joint pain (because other NSAIDs are avoided in these patients due to risk of bleeding).

NSaids should be taken daily and with food to lessen stomach upset or heart burn (a burning sensation in the middle of the chest). You may need to avoid foods and beverages, including alcohol, that irritate the lining of your stomach and esophagus (the tube that carries swallowed food and liquid to the stomach). This results from impairment of the function of the sphincter between your stomach and esophagus. You should avoid lying down within 2 hours after eating, stop smoking, if you are a smoker. You may need to raise the head of your bed about 6 inches (15 cm) when sleeping. It is wise to lose weight if you are overweight.

There is an increased risk of GI bleeding from ulcers, especially among people over the age of 60, or those who have a previous history of peptic ulcer disease. If you have any acute abdominal pain, severe cramps or burning, vomiting, diarrhea, or black tarry stools, seek medical attention promptly. Some NSAIDs, in particular indomethacin, can cause headache, drowsiness, and some impairment of cognitive functions (a "spaced-out" feeling), especially in elderly people.

NSAIDs should not be used for chest pain resulting from coronary heart disease, and their chronic use by elderly people may, unlike low-dose aspirin, increase their risk of heart attack or stroke. Some individuals are allergic to NSAIDs and develop skin rash or, more seriously, shortness of breath, especially among people with asthma. Such patients are also more likely to be allergic to some of the other NSAIDs as well.

How do they work?

There are chemical compounds called prostaglandins, produced in the body by the enzymes called cyclooxygenases (COX) that serve important functions, including promotion of inflammation to facilitate healing from infection or injury. This healing process also results in pain, fever, and other effects. COX enzymes exist in two forms, COX-1 and COX-2. COX-1 can be considered the "good enzyme" because it helps in keeping intact the lining of the stomach and duodenum, and maintaining normal flow of blood through the kidneys and normal platelet stickiness and aggregation. If not enough COX-1 is produced or its function is inhibited, the intestinal lining becomes vulnerable to ulceration and there may also be impairment of kidney and platelet function. COX-2 is one of the important enzymes responsible for pain and inflammation when it is produced in access due to infection, injury, or arthritis.

COX-2 inhibitors

They are a type of NSAIDs that selectively target cyclooxygenase-2 (COX-2) enzyme, unlike the conventional NSAIDs that are non-selective in this regard. Celecoxib (Celebrex®) is the only COX-2-specific (or -selective) NSAID currently available in the US. Rofecoxib (Vioxx®), etoricoxib (Arcoxia®), and valdecoxib (Bextra®), as mentioned earlier, are not available in the US. However, COX-2 inhibitors are no more effective than the conventional NSAIDs, and like them, may cause fluid retention, some increase in blood pressure or potential impairment of kidney function. But celecoxib (Celebrex®) carries a lower risk of peptic ulceration (stomach and duodenal ulcers) and resultant bleeding due to sparing of the COX-1 enzyme.

Conventional DMARDs

The drugs sulfasalazine and methotrexate are called conventional DMARDs (disease modifying anti-rheumatic drugs), and therefore the abbreviations c-DMARDs, or sometimes called synthetic DMARDs (s-DMARDs), or conventional synthetic DMARDs (cs-DMARDs). These prefixes in lower case are frequently used to distinguish them from the b-DMARDs such as the biologic drugs such as TNF inhibitors. The cs-DMARDs are also called slow-acting anti-rheumatic drugs (SAARDs) because any benefit from these drugs takes some time to manifest. Unlike NSAIDs, they are not pain relievers but they will help relieve pain if they can first heal or control the underlying inflammation.

Sulfasalazine and methotrexate may have some short-term benefit for AS patients with peripheral arthritis or concomitant IBD. Treatment with sulfasalazine does reduce the risk of recurrences of acute uveitis in patients with AS. But since the availability of b-DMARDs, such as TNF inhibitors and IL-17 inhibitors, the use of the c-DMARDs is not advised for typical AS patients with spinal involvement, but they are still being used in less-developed countries because of either lack of availability or high cost of the biologics.

19

Tumor Necrosis Factor inhibitors

 Key points

- During the last 2 decades, increasingly more effective drugs have become available for treatment of patients who fail to adequately respond to NSAIDs. They are grouped under the term "biologics," "biologicals," or "biologic disease-modifying anti-rheumatic drugs" (b-DMARDs).

- Biologics are produced by using biotechnology that requires living microorganisms or animal or human cells, or components of living organisms.

- They include TNF inhibitors, the subject of this chapter, and IL-17 and IL-23 inhibitors, discussed in the next chapter, and many others that are used for other disease.

- Biologics do not cure arthritis and will help only if you continue taking them at the recommended dose.

- The most recent data indicate that there is slowing down of progression of AS/axSpA that becomes noticeable on X-ray 2 to 4 years after initiation of treatment with TNF inhibitors, especially if the treatment is initiated in early stages of the disease.

- TNF-inhibitors are generally well tolerated, but you need to discuss with your healthcare providers and pharmacists, the most common as well as potentially serious adverse effects.

Ankylosing Spondylitis and Axial Spondyloarthritis, Second Edition. Muhammad Asim Khan, Oxford University Press.
© Oxford University Press 2023. DOI: 10.1093/oso/9780198864158.003.0019

Introduction

Non-steroidal anti-inflammatory drugs (NSAIDs) are first line treatment but the response can be inadequate, or over time there is loss of efficacy. Thus, there was an unmet need for AS/axSpA patients whose disease cannot be controlled with conventional therapy. Luckily, during the last 2 decades, increasingly more effective drugs have become available for such patients. They are grouped under the term "biologic disease-modifying anti-rheumatic drugs" (b-DMARDs), such as the TNF inhibitors, and, more recently, inhibitors of another inflammatory proteins (cytokines) named interleukin-17 (IL-17) and IL-23.

What is a biologic?

Biological drugs or simply "biologics" are produced by using biotechnology that requires living microorganisms or animal or human cells, or components of living organisms. They are therefore harder to produce under strict quality control and are thus much more costly.

What is TNF?

TNF stands for Tumor Necrosis Factor, and it is one of many messenger proteins called cytokines that play a key role in the body's immune defenses and interact with many other molecular structures to achieve that result. The effect of TNF is to promote inflammation and to help cells heal or repair themselves. It attaches to a cell surface protein called TNF receptor on the cells belonging to the immune system. This surface receptor draws TNF into the cell for it to exert its effect. When cells have enough TNF, they release from their surface some of their TNF receptors into the bloodstream. These released TNF receptors mop up any excess TNF that is circulating in the bloodstream or is present in the tissues.

The original reason for calling this substance "tumor necrosis factor" was that it could induce destruction (necrosis) of cancerous tumors in laboratory studies. It was later tested for its ability to induce destruction of cancerous tumors in animals. Later when it was tested in cancer patients, the doses needed to shrink tumors were too large and caused serious toxic reactions.

What are TNF inhibitors?

If too much TNF is produced in the body, it can damage healthy tissues and contribute to a variety of ailments, such as RA and AS. The first TNF inhibitor is named *infliximab* (trade name Remicade®) is a bioengineered hybrid molecule (made by combining human and mouse proteins) that snags and neutralizes excess TNF and keeps it from binding to its receptors on cell surfaces. The original human trial of this TNF inhibitor to treat RA was started in 1992, and the FDA in the US approved its use to treat RA in 1999. It had earlier been approved in 1998 for the treatment of CD, and has subsequently been approved for treating patients with AS, PsA, psoriasis, and both adult and pediatric UC (Table 19.1). It is given by intravenous infusion at the doctor's office.

A genetically engineered and human-derived molecule called *etanercept* (Enbrel®) has a similar anti-TNF effect. It is composed of components of the normal human TNF receptor attached to a normal human blood immunoglobulin protein called IgG1. It acts as a decoy TNF receptor that snags and neutralizes excess TNF and keeps it from binding the TNF receptors on cell surfaces. Etanercept is injected under the skin (subcutaneous injection), and patients can easily learn how to inject themselves.

Infliximab and etanercept were the first two TNF inhibitors, and subsequently, others have been developed and the list now includes *adalimumab* (Humira®), *golimumab* (Simponi®), and *certolizumab* (Cimzia®). With the exception of etanercept, these are all monoclonal antibodies that specifically target TNF. All TNF inhibitors show similarity in their efficacy in treating AS/axSpA and some of other forms of SpA, without the need for concomitant use of methotrexate, sulfasalazine, or other cs-DMARDs. Etanercept, unlike the monoclonal TNF inhibitors, is not effective in treating IBD, and is also less effective in preventing recurrent episodes of acute anterior uveitis.

Most patients show quite a rapid and remarkable improvement in the patients' symptoms and signs, including back pain and stiffness, and arthritis in the extremities. They also improve HR-QoL, PROM, sleep quality, fatigue, anemia, and bone density. Clinical improvement is accompanied by a significant decrease in inflammation, as evidenced by a dramatic reduction in the level of inflammation as detected by measuring CRP and ESR. Sustained disease remission is more likely in patients attaining normalized CRP.

Recent data indicate that there is slowing down of X-ray progression that becomes noticeable 2 to 4 years of sustained remission after initiation of the treatment with TNF inhibitors. Some patients may not respond or lose efficacy with time. Treatment efficacy and retention rates are lower among female patients initiating their first TNF inhibitors. Switching to an alternative TNF inhibitor or increasing the dose or frequency of administration may sometimes overcome this problem. The choice of TNF inhibitor should be guided by the presence of the arthritis and other associated manifestations, and the patient's preference because of differences in mode of administration.

Table 19.1 List of TNF inhibitors approved in the US (by FDA) that also shows their approved indication

FDA-approved TNF Inhibitors	Infliximab	Etanercept	Adalimumab	Certolizumab	Golimumab
RA	✓	✓	✓	✓	✓
AS	✓	✓	✓	✓	✓
PsA	✓	✓	✓	✓	✓
Plaque psoriasis	✓	✓	✓	✓	
Ulcerative colitis	✓		✓		✓
Adult Crohn's disease	✓		✓	✓	
Pediatric Crohn's disease	✓		✓		
Hydradenitis suppurativa			✓		✓
Juvenile idiopathic arthritis (polyarticular)		✓	✓		
Uveitis (intermediate, posterior, or panuveitis)			✓		
nr-axSpA				✓	

Response to TNF inhibitors may be sustained over several years, but symptoms almost invariably return due to disease flare-up when this therapy is completely stopped. Men in general show a somewhat better response than women. Obese and overweight patients and smokers have a lower response rate to TNF inhibitors and have a worse outcome. Because of the high cost of long-term treatment, some of the more recent studies have shown that good disease control has been maintained with widening the interval between the injections or a reduction in the dose in some patient. The most recent studies report that after 2 years of clinical disease remission, approximately 50% of patients had successfully decreased the dose of their TNF inhibitors, but it could be permanently discontinued in only 1% of the patients.

Potential untoward effects

TNF inhibitors are generally well tolerated, with the common adverse effects being minor and transient, not needing drug discontinuation. A large majority of these adverse effects are upper respiratory tract infections like nasal congestion and runny nose, sinusitis, cough, and pharyngitis. You need to discuss with your healthcare providers and pharmacists, the most common as well as potentially serious adverse effects of TNF inhibitors. There can be injection-site reactions from injection under the skin, and infusion reactions with the intravenous route of administration.

TNF is broadly involved in body's immune defenses, and therefore its targeting by TNF inhibitors may impair the immune system's capacity to mount protective responses against certain infections. There is a potential risk of opportunistic infections and reactivation of some of the pre-existing infections that can be bacterial (including tuberculosis (TB)), fungal (e.g., histoplasmosis), or viral (e.g., hepatitis B and C). Patients should talk to their rheumatologist before getting any vaccinations, and live vaccines should be avoided. All patients should receive pneumococcal and shingles (herpes zoster) vaccines before starting TNF inhibitor therapy. Yearly influenza vaccination is advised, as well as proper vaccination against COVID-19. More severe COVID-19 outcomes in patients suffering from AS/axSpA are not due to the TNF inhibitor use but largely due to older age, obesity, diabetes and other comorbid conditions, and use of some of the other immunosuppressants.

A patient with a positive screening test for TB may need to be treated according to country-specific guidelines. Physicians need to monitor the patients for any untoward effects, including signs and symptoms of active bacterial, viral, or fungal infections, and therefore continued surveillance remains imperative. Patients living in areas with a higher incidence of certain fungal infections such as coccidioidomycosis or histoplasmosis should have screening for these conditions before initiating therapy with TNF inhibitors. Treatment should be withheld in patients who develop a serious infection or sepsis until it is resolved.

Use in pregnancy

Women in their child-bearing years need to discuss with their physician about the safety of these medications in pregnancy and during lactation. TNF inhibitors do not cross the placenta until the end of the second trimester. Their use in pregnancy should be a consideration only if there is a clear and strong indication. Use of certolizumab pegol (Cimzia®) is approved for use during pregnancy because it differs from other TNF inhibitors in that it is not actively transported through the placenta, and therefore its concentrations in the fetus would be much lower. Moreover, its presence in the mother's breast milk will be lower. If approved by your treating rheumatologist, monoclonal TNF-inhibitors infliximab, adalimumab, and golimumab should be discontinued around 20th week of pregnancy, and etanercept may be continued until week 30–32.

What is a biosimilar?

A biosimilar is a biologic product "highly similar" to another already approved biologic, and these have the same standards of pharmaceutical quality, safety, and efficacy. They are subsequent versions of biologic made by a different pharmaceutical company following patent expiration on the innovator product. A biological product may be demonstrated to be "biosimilar" if the manufacturer can provide evidence that shows that, among other things, their product is "highly similar" to an already-approved biological product. But the two products are not considered interchangeable and are therefore not called generics. Biosimilars provide comparable clinical results to innovator biologics but at a lower cost. Some of the early examples of FDA approved biosimilars include Inflectra® (infliximab-dyyb), which is a biosimilar for Remicade®, and Erelzi® (etanercept-sass), a biosimilar for Enbrel®. Because of the high cost of long-term treatment, an annual tender system was introduced in Norway in 2008, and that has resulted in an approximately 50% reduction in the cost of biologics over subsequent years in that country.

Storage of biologics and other medications

Biologics are protein molecules that require special storage that needs to be meticulously followed. You need to work closely with your physician, nurse, and pharmacist to make sure that you know not only how to self-inject but also how to store the medications. The manufacture and expiry dates are shown on the bottle or container when you buy any medicines. As a rule, discard medicines when they reach their expiry date or which have not been stored properly. Keep all medications out of reach of children, even if the bottles have "child-resistant" caps, because these caps are not "child proof." The medications that do not require refrigeration should not be stored in the bathroom cabinet because humidity and heat may impair their effectiveness.

20

IL-17 and IL-23 inhibitors and targeted synthetic DMARDs

 Key points

- Many novel drugs are being developed that have further revolutionized the care of patients with SpA, especially for patients who fail to respond to TNF inhibitors.

- IL-17 inhibitors secukinumab (Cosentyx®) and ixekizumab (Taltz®) are very effective for the treatment of patients with active AS/axSpA, psoriasis, and PsA, but they are not effective for IBD.

- The most recent data indicate that there is slowing down of X-ray progression of AS/axSpA that becomes noticeable a couple of years after initiation of treatment with IL-17 inhibitors, if the treatment is initiated in early stages of the disease.

- IL-23 inhibitors ustekinumab (Stelara®), guselkumab (Tremfya®) and risankizumab (Skyrizi®) are approved for psoriasis and PsA. They have unprecedented efficacy of even complete skin clearance of psoriasis in a high percentage of patients, as compared to TNF inhibitors. But they are not effective for patients with AS/axSpA.

- Tofactinib (Xeljanz®) and upadacitinib (Rinvoq®) are non-biologic drugs called JAK inhibitors that are taken as a tablet and have been approved for the treatment of AS and PsA. Tofactinib is also approved for the treatment of UC and upadacitinib for nr-axSpA. They belong to a class of drugs called targeted synthetic DMARDs (ts-DMARDs).

♦ Apremilast (Otezla®), a non-biologic drug belonging to PDE4 (phosphodiesterase 4) inhibitors, is approved for the treatment of psoriasis and PsA.

Introduction

As has been discussed earlier, NSAIDs still provide the first line of treatment, and the introduction of TNFi was a great advance. However, some patients do not respond to them or have an inadequate or gradually diminishing response. That has led to the use of a newer biologics that target other pro-inflammatory protein molecules (cytokines), such as interleukin-23 (IL-23) and IL-17. A dysregulation of the so-called IL-23/IL-17 axis results in excessive production of these cytokines, in addition to that of TNF. During the COVID-19 pandemic, it is reassuring to know that use of none of the drugs discussed in this chapter seem to be associated with severe COVID-19 outcomes. The worst outcome is largely driven by old age, obesity and comorbid condition, like diabetes, or the use of some of the other immunosuppressant drugs.

IL-17 inhibitors

IL-17 is a pro-inflammatory cytokine that plays a critical role, along with the above-mentioned cytokines, in tissue repair and immune response for protection against bacterial and fungal microbial invasion of the barrier surfaces of the gut and the skin. But when produced in excess, IL-17 can contribute to occurrence of various inflammatory diseases, including psoriasis, AS, and related forms of SpA. This knowledge had made IL-17 an attractive treatment target.

IL-17-inhibitor secukinumab (Cosentyx®), a fully human monoclonal antibody, and ixekizumab (Taltz®), a "humanized" monoclonal antibody, have now been approved for the treatment of psoriasis, PsA, AS, and nr-axSpA. The most recent data indicate that there is slowing down of X-ray progression of AS/axSpA that becomes noticeable a couple of years after initiation of treatment with IL-17-inhibitors, especially if the treatment is initiated in early stages of the disease. But they, unlike monoclonal TNF-inhibitors, are not effective for treating IBD, and, on rare occasions, can even activate IBD. This necessitates monitoring for signs and symptoms of IBD in patients on treatment with IL-17-inhibitors. These biologics also do not decrease the risk of occurrence of acute uveitis.

Secukinumab (Cosentyx®) and ixekizumab (Taltz®) are administered by injection under the skin (subcutaneous). Redness, pain, and tenderness for a couple of days after the injection (often called injection site reaction) is very uncommon with secukinumab but can occur in roughly 10% of patient on ixekizumab (Taltz®), although its occurrence recedes with subsequent injections. Secukinumab (Cosentyx®) can be given without or with a loading dose at weeks 0, 1, 2, 3, and 4, and every 4 weeks thereafter. Ixekizumab (Taltz®) is given once every 4 weeks.

They, like TNF inhibitors and many other biologics, can increase the risk of infections. Caution should be exercised when considering their use in patients with a chronic infection or a history of recurrent infection. If a serious infection develops, treatment should be discontinued until the infection resolves. The infections usually affect upper respiratory tract, such as nasopharyngitis (the common cold), and are usually mild and respond to treatment. Candida infection in mucous lining such as in the throat (thrush) can occur (1.2% with secukinumab versus 0.3% on placebo control subjects). It resolves spontaneously or with standard antifungal treatment, without the need for discontinuation of treatment with IL-17 inhibitors.

Brodalumab (Siliq®) is another IL-17 inhibitor, but it is only approved for the treatment of psoriasis. Of note, it carries in its label a "black box" warning about potential "suicidal behavior and ideation." Lastly, bimekizumab is a first-of-its-kind dual IL-17 inhibitor because it targets both IL-17A and IL-17 F cytokines, and ongoing clinical studies have shown promising initial results in treating patients with psoriasis, AS, and nr-axSpA. But in May 2022, FDA did not approve the drug manufacturer's request for approval for its use to treat psoriasis.

IL-23 inhibitors

Ustekinumab (Stelara®) is an IL-12/IL-23 inhibitor approved for the treatment of psoriasis, PsA, and IBD (both UC and CD), and IL-23 inhibitors guselkumab (Tremfya®) and risankizumab (Skyrizi®) are approved for psoriasis and PsA. These have unprecedented efficacy of even complete skin clearance of psoriasis in a high percentage of patients, as compared to the TNF inhibitors. However, they are not effective in the treatment of AS/axSpA. Another IL-23 inhibitors, tidrakizumab (Ilumya®) is approved only for the treatment of psoriasis. Please see Chapter 10 for further discussion on IL-23 inhibitors and management of PsA and IBD.

Targeted synthetic DMARDs

Janus kinase (JAK) inhibitors

When cytokines attach to their receptors on a cell of the immune system, a signal is sent to the cell to make more cytokines via activation of intracellular protein molecules called Janus Kinases or JAKs that are a set of enzymes labelled JAK-1, JAK-2, JAK-3, and TYK-2. They transmit this signal from the cell membrane downstream within the cell to produce more cytokines. Thus, the JAK signaling pathway plays an important role in promotion of inflammation by release of inflammatory cytokines. For example, they are involved in the IL-23/IL-17 pathway.

JAK inhibitors (JAKinibs or JAKi for short) are small molecules that have been synthesized to inhibit the JAK signaling pathway. They are taken by mouth once or twice daily in a tablet form and are grouped under the term targeted synthetic DMARDs or ts-DMARDs for short. They are not biologics, are less costly to make, carry no risks of anti-drug antibody formation, and do not require special storage. But they should not be given in combination with biologics. Tofacitinib (Xeljanz®), the first JAK inhibitor, is approved for the treatment of adults with active AS, PsA, and UC. Upadacitinib (Rinvoq®), another JAK inhibitor, has been approved for the treatment of adults with active nr-axSpA, AS, and PsA.

JAK inhibitors have narrow window of efficacy and safety, and they carry a warning on their label regarding possible injury and death because of many potential untoward effects, such as blood clots and venous thromboembolic events, heart attacks, infections, shingles, lymphomas, and other malignancies. In September 2021 the US FDA mandated a "black box" warning that states that tofacitinib and upadacitinib increase the risk of thromboembolic events and malignancy. To decrease the risk of shingles (herpes zoster), injection of a vaccine named Shingrix® is advised, preferably 2–4 weeks prior to initiation of therapy. This is particularly important in elderly and immune-compromised patients, people with a prior history of shingles, and those with Asian ancestry.

Baricitinib (Olumiant®) is another JAK inhibitor; it blocks JAK-1 and JAK-2 but also carries the above-mentioned black box warning. It has been approved for the treatment of RA but not AS. It is of interest that WHO has approved its use to treat COVID-19 patients, and it does not need to be co-administered with remdesivir, another approved drug for this disease.

Phosphodiesterase 4 (PDE4) inhibitors

These are also small molecules, not biologics, and are taken by mouth in a tablet form. Apremilast (Otezla®) is one of the PDE4 inhibitors that is approved only for the treatment of psoriasis and PsA but is not effective in the treatment of AS/axSpA.

21

Living with the disease and its socio-economic impact

 Key points

- Most people with AS/axSpA can cope well and continue to have a very productive and active lifestyle, especially with the advent of more effective drug therapies and earlier diagnosis of their disease.

- They can mostly maintain some level of employment even in manual and semi-skilled types of work. Some patients, especially those with severe AS with complete spinal fusion and physically demanding jobs, may need to change their type of work, decrease their work hours, or experience temporary work disability and even loss of their employment.

- Occupational therapists can be very helpful in making the employer aware of the patient-specific physical limitations and needs. They can also come up with necessary work adaptations agreeable with the employer.

- Looking physically different from the rest of the population can present psychological problems, but most people are able to come to terms with this.

- Most of the socio-economic factors associated with higher cost are related to uncontrolled disease activity and functional disability.

- Therefore, early appropriate treatment is crucial, and interventions that maintain or improve patients' functional ability are likely to have the greatest potential to decrease the costs of AS.

Introduction

Most people with AS/axSpA can cope well and continue to have a very productive and active lifestyle, especially with the advent of more effective drug

Ankylosing Spondylitis and Axial Spondyloarthritis, Second Edition. Muhammad Asim Khan, Oxford University Press.
© Oxford University Press 2023. DOI: 10.1093/oso/9780198864158.003.0021

therapies and earlier diagnosis of their disease. Patients are capable of performing various jobs, and many have had very successful and productive business and professional careers. In most cases patients can get life insurance and mortgages for purchasing a home in economically developed nations. They can maintain the level of employment in manual and semi-skilled types of work. Some patients, especially those with severe AS with complete spinal fusion and physically demanding jobs, may need to change their type of work, decrease their work hours, or experience temporary work disability and possible job loss. Patients with contracture of the hip joints have benefitted tremendously from hip joint replacement. Spinal fusion, if accompanied by forward stooping of neck and curvature in the upper back, can make it difficult to even look straight ahead. Looking physically different from the rest of the population can present psychological problems, but most people are able to come to terms with this.

Patient experiences and perspectives are highlighted by the results of the recent European Mapping of Axial Spondyloarthritis (EMAS) Survey of 2,486 patients living with AS/axSpA from 13 European countries has recently been published. It is discussed later in this chapter. An older study of 100 people with AS in Norway reported that just over half were employed in full-time work after a mean disease duration of 16 years. All of this has a tremendous impact on patients and on society at large in terms of economic costs, both direct healthcare and non-healthcare costs. Moreover, unlike RA, AS usually begins at the prime of one's life, so these patients must deal with the illness for a longer time. Early cessation of employment for patients with AS is associated not only with physically demanding jobs, but also occurs more often among people with low level of education, complete fusion of the spine (bamboo spine), hip joint involvement, eye inflammation (acute anterior uveitis), and coexistence of nonrheumatic diseases. Cost of illness studies classically analyze the direct healthcare and non-healthcare costs, productivity costs, and intangible costs. Functional disability is usually the most important predictor of high total costs.

A study has shown presence of remarkable differences in work status and productivity costs between three neighboring European countries. This has implications for the generalizability of health economic studies, and there are limitations of comparability of cost of illness studies that have been published. Direct healthcare costs alone do not describe the total costs associated with AS, and the productivity losses associated with AS are considerable. Most of the factors associated with higher cost were related to greater disease activity and functional disability. Therefore, early appropriate treatment is crucial, and interventions that maintain or improve patients' functional ability are likely to have the greatest potential to decrease the costs of AS. TNF and IL-17 inhibitors are highly effective in AS in alleviating pain and reducing clinical disease activity, reducing or alleviating extraarticular manifestations such as eye inflammation, psoriasis, and IBD, improving quality of life, and maintaining long-term efficacy. The clinical response is greater in patients with earlier stages of disease and less damage.

The increasingly availability of the much more effective therapies, early diagnosis, and early initiation of such treatment is improving continuous employability of patients with AS and related forms of SpA. But the ability to undertake productive work is influenced by the type of occupation, the patient's lifestyle, as well as social, cultural, and emotional factors. Therefore understanding these potential risk factors may further contribute to the development of preventive strategies to maintain patient participation in the labor force. These considerations, together with the convincing evidence that effective but expensive treatments sustain improvements in work outcomes, have resulted in socio-economic benefits for the patients and the society in general.

There is a need to inculcate in all patients with chronic rheumatic diseases a positive type of coping response for dealing with health and daily-life stressors. This can result in better outcomes than those adopting negative or evasive strategies to cope with their disease and emotional responses that reflect poor adjustment to disease. Patients using positive coping mechanisms generally have good social as well as family relationships, a good educational level, and stable jobs. The negative type of coping is generally associated with low educational level, poor health outcomes, and the individual's independent social role; and it results in low health status, high level of pain, low adherence to treatment, and long-term risk behavior.

Health-related quality of life

Health-related quality of life is based on your perception of the net effects an illness has on your life. It is commonly based on your symptoms, physical functioning, ability to work, psychosocial functioning and interaction, untoward effects of treatment, and direct and indirect medical and financial costs. Although people with AS are troubled with pain, stiffness, and limited spinal mobility, most of them remain in employment.

In a survey of 175 AS patients (68% male, mean disease duration of 23.7 years, mean age 51 years), the most common quality of life concern was about stiffness (90%), pain (83%), fatigue (62%), poor sleep (54%), appearance (51%), side-effects of medications (41%), and concern about the future (50%). Few patients in this survey reported problems with social relations or mood.

The much larger EMAS survey mentioned earlier, comprised 2,846 patients with a diagnosis of AS (79.2%), nr-axSpA (8.5%), or just axSpA without specifying the subtype (12.3%). HLA-B27 tested positive in 71% of those who reported their HLA-B27 status. Their mean age was 44 years, 61% females, age of symptom onset was 26 years, mean disease duration of 17 years, mean delay of diagnosis 7.4 years, and 76% reported moderate to severe spinal stiffness throughout the day. Around 20% of participants reported a diagnosis of an extra-articular manifestation, comprising uveitis or IBD. Their daily life was substantially impaired: 74% reported difficulties finding a job due to the disease, and 61.5% reported psychological distress, with 1 out of 3 reporting anxiety and/or depression. Nearly half of the participants reported that their disease influenced their job choice and 74% had difficulties finding a job due to the disease. Participants commonly reported fear of disease progression or loss of mobility and hoping for a more effective treatment that will halt disease progression and eliminate pain. However, one-third of the participants surveyed reported that they had not talked to their clinician about their personal treatment goals.

Depression

Depression is not uncommon in people with any chronic painful illness that impairs quality of life, and that includes AS. Depression is a treatable disease that has many underlying causes, and some individuals are genetically more prone to it. Symptoms of depression include:

♦ loss of pleasure in activities that were once enjoyable

♦ persistent feeling of sadness, emptiness, decreased energy, tiredness, and anxiety

♦ frequently feeling helpless, worthless, guilty, and hopeless, or feeling irritable and restless

♦ disturbed appetite (loss of appetite or tendency to overeat)

♦ disturbed sleep (difficulty sleeping, waking up too early, oversleeping, sleeping too little or too much)

♦ difficulty in concentrating, thinking, remembering, or decision-making

♦ sometimes persistent physical problems (e.g., headache, abdominal pain) not responding to treatment

♦ thoughts of ending life by committing suicide

If you have any of these symptoms, you should discuss them with your doctor and allied health professionals so that appropriate treatment can be provided. Additional information on depression is available from the National Institute of Mental Health (<http://www.nimh.nih.gov>) or the American Psychiatric Association (<http://www.psych.org>).

Posture

People with AS always need to practice good posture habits and should be taught about dynamic, resting, and occupational postures. A daily routine of deep breathing exercises at frequent intervals during the day, along with spine motion/stretching exercises may minimize the fusion, and at least preserve better posture. Be aware of how you are standing, try to maintain an erect and tall posture, with the spine kept as straight as possible, and avoid any tendency to slump forward. Proper sitting, sleeping, walking, and working positions, coupled with appropriate exercises, help maintain good posture and chest expansion. Avoid using low, soft sofas to sit on because they will worsen back pain and stiffness, and can, over the years, lead to bad posture. Because hip and shoulder joints are often affected, you should exercise the range of motion of these joints even before you observe any symptoms or limited motion there.

It is important to sleep on a firm bed to maintain a good resting posture at night. Avoid a saggy mattress or a waterbed. A suitable board (made of plywood

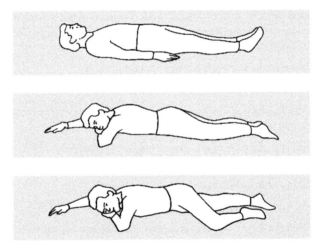

Figure 21.1 Recommended sleeping positions: A flat sleeping position on a firm bed opposes the tendency of curvature. If your head would fall into over-extension because your thoracic spine is already curved, a small pillow of just the right thickness under the back of your head may make the position easier. Avoid too thick a pillow. Lying "face down" ("on your stomach") is also a favorable position, and if it is no longer possible, lying on your side is a good alternative.

Reprinted with kind permission from Morbus Bechterew—ein Leitfaden für Patienten, by Ernst Feldtkeller, Deutsche Vereinigung Morbus Bechterew (DVMB), Schweinfurt, 1985.

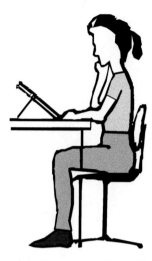

Figure 21.2 Proper sitting and working position with straight back and occupying the entire seat of the chair with back support, and working with a tilting work surface on the table.

Reprinted with kind permission from Morbus Bechterew—ein Leitfaden für Patienten, by Ernst Feldtkeller, Novartis Pharma Verlag, Nürnberg, 1997.

or chipboard) can be put between the mattress and the bed frame to make the bed firmer. You should preferably make a habit of sleeping on your back, to prevent the hip joints and the back from becoming bent (Figure 21.1a). Avoid using a pillow if possible or use one just thick enough to allow a horizontal position of the face to prevent pain from overextension of the neck. Also avoid a pillow under your knees because that will increase the tendency to muscle and tendon shortening. You should only lie on your side for short periods, if possible. You should also practice lying prone (with the face down), for example for 5 minutes or more before getting out of the bed in the morning, and before going to bed at night (Figure 21.1 b and c), or you can lie on your back across your bed with your legs over the side and knees bent.

You should regularly perform appropriate muscle-strengthening exercises advised by your doctor. Splints, braces, and corsets are not helpful and are not advised. Some form of bracing may be necessary on rare occasions, for example after injury to the back or neck, but only on the recommendation of a doctor who is experienced in the management of AS patients.

It may be necessary to modify your working positions to maintain a good posture. For example, a drafting table with tilting work surface (Figure 21.2) may

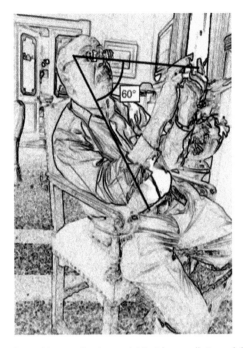

Figure 21.3 A patient with severely advanced AS with a totally immobile spine, including his neck, and severely limited mobility of his hip joints is sitting in a crooked position on a chair, occupying only the front of the seat. He was able to thereby acquire approximately 60 degree angle to enable him to obtain a picture with a full panoramic view by using his cell phone. He is not able to take such a picture while sitting back and occupying the entire seat because his hip arthritis would not allow it.

be better than an ordinary office desk for writing and reading and avoiding stress on your neck. However, if you have completely fused (ankylosed) spine and restricted ability to bend you hip joints, the reality often looks quite different. The patient in Figure 21.3 with advanced AS (with ankylosed spine and immobile and forwardly stooped neck) and marked limitation of mobility of his hip joints, is sitting on the front edge of the chair in order to achieve a straight (horizonal) position of his vision to take a picture with a panoramic view by his cellphone.

Avoid physical activity that places prolonged strain on your back and neck muscles, and prolonged stooping or bending. Alternate between sitting and standing positions to perform jobs that take a long time to finish. Be aware of your posture and try to correct it constantly. Avoid heavy lifts, and never lift and turn at the same time. During your midday break at work, lie face down on a firm surface for a few minutes, and stretch your back. (Figure 21.1 b, and c). Occupational therapists can be very helpful in making the employer aware of your specific physical limitations and needs. They can also come up with necessary work adaptations agreeable with the employer.

Family and sex life

People living with AS generally have a very fulfilling and productive life and raise children just like anyone else. Fertility, pregnancy, and childbirth is usually normal, and children grow up normally. A short story with graphics titled "Dad has Ankylosing Spondylitis" is available on the website of the Canadian Spondylitis Association (<http://www.spondylitis.ca>) that is very useful for AS patients to explain their illness to their children. The disease usually starts at the prime and sexually most active period of one's life. Sometimes family, social, and sex life may be impacted because of severe back pain and stiffness, fatigue, impaired spinal mobility and/or deformity, or severe hip joint involvement. These aspects and some misunderstandings can put strain on a loving relationship and patients may need sexual counseling. The pain and impaired mobility of the hip joints can respond to THR surgery (see Chapter 23 and Figure 23.1). You should also freely discuss these problems with your healthcare providers.

Useful and informative brochures that discuss housework, dressing and grooming, sexual intimacy, childbearing, and childcare are available from national patients' societies of various countries affiliated with Axial Spondyloarthritis International Federation (<http://www.ASIF.info/en>). They are highly recommended for additional information and advice. The Spondylitis Association of America (<http://www.spondylitis.org>) is one such US affiliate of ASIF that has published a booklet titled *Straight Talk on Spondylitis*, and it is also available online. Similar materials are also available from many other patient self-help groups or societies in many other countries. See Appendix 1 for contact details.

Women with AS can have children and pregnancy does not provide any special concerns either for the mother or baby. Birth takes place by the normal route, but a Caesarian section may sometimes be needed, especially if there is severe hip joint involvement. Pregnancy does not usually affect the symptoms of AS but there may be restrictions on the use of certain kinds of drug therapy during pregnancy and breastfeeding. Certolizumab pegol (Cimzia is its brand name) is the TNF inhibitor that can be continued during pregnancy as it does not cross the placenta and therefore the fetus is not exposed to the drug. You should discuss the use of any drug at these times with your doctor. The growth and development of infants and young children seem to be comparable to those of other mothers unaffected by AS.

Driving cars and other automobiles

Driving for a long distance may worsen back pain and stiffness, and you may need to stop at rest places and get out of the car to walk around and do back stretching exercises. Avoid using "bucket' seats and choose adjustable seats with good back and neck support. Always use seatbelts and head restraints so that sudden slowing or stoppage does not jerk the spine, especially the neck. Remember that the stiff neck of an AS patient is more vulnerable to injury than a normal neck. The top of the car seat's head restraint should be level with the top of your head, and the restraint should be adjustable to bring it as close to the back of your head as possible.

You may find difficulty driving if you have impaired mobility of your neck. It may also make it difficult to you to change gear with a "stick shift" if you cannot look down, necessitating use of cars that have automatic gear shifts. The limitation in turning and twisting your neck and back may make it difficult for you to reverse the car into tight parking spaces. Special wide-view mirrors and/or cameras can be installed in your car, but you will need some practice sessions driving and reversing the car in an open area to become comfortable using them. A small hand-held mirror may be of use in special situations in avoiding tight corners and 'blind spots." If you can afford. the newest autonomous car models, with automated assist devices and cameras are the best for you. A disabled driver's parking permit is appropriate if you cannot walk very far or need a wider parking space. Useful booklets are available from ASIF and its affiliates worldwide; see Appendix 1 for contact details.

22

Fused (ankylosed) spine and risk of fractures

> ## ➲ Key points
>
> ◆ Structural deterioration due to net bone loss (osteoporosis), along with spinal immobility due to bony fusion, make the spine fragile and very susceptible to fractures, both post-traumatic as well as spontaneous vertebral compression fracture.
>
> ◆ These structural changes, as well as associated weakness of the muscles around the spine, problems with keeping balance, and decreasing field of view due to forward stooping and immobile neck, further increase susceptibility to spinal fractures.
>
> ◆ The spinal fracture usually occurs in the cervical spine, and neurologic deficits are often subtle on initial presentation, resulting in the fracture being missed because of a low index of suspicion and poor visualization of lower cervical fractures on conventional X-rays. MRI or CT scan results may be more helpful in confirming or excluding such spinal fractures.
>
> ◆ Patients with AS/axSpA or anyone with limited neck or spinal mobility should also avoid manipulation of their back or neck by chiropractors and masseurs because such treatments have sometimes inadvertently led to spinal fractures and neurological complications.
>
> ◆ Availability of biologics has greatly enhanced the treatment, and a few observational studies have shown that long term use of biologics may slow down new bone formation that results in spinal ankylosis.

Ankylosing Spondylitis and Axial Spondyloarthritis, Second Edition. Muhammad Asim Khan, Oxford University Press.
© Oxford University Press 2023. DOI: 10.1093/oso/9780198864158.003.0022

Introduction

Our understanding of molecular mechanisms leading to new bone formation in AS/axSpA has significantly improved but there are still many unanswered questions. Availability of biologics has greatly enhanced the treatment, and, as mentioned at other places in this book, a few observational studies have shown that long term use of biologics may slow down new bone formation that binds adjacent vertebral bodies of patients with progressive disease. The patients also develop net loss of bone (porous bone called osteoporosis) in the spine, and that can occur relatively early in the disease course, possibly due to high disease activity with increased level of proinflammatory cytokines and an alteration in vitamin D metabolism. A marked reduction in bone mineral density of the lumbar spine and femoral neck has been observed on DEXA measurement to detect osteoporosis (see Chapter 20), even in relatively young patients with AS. These structural changes in patients with ankylosed spine are often associated with progressive weakness of the muscles surrounding the spinal column, and problems with keeping balance. Moreover, decreasing field of view due to forward stooping and immobile neck further increase susceptibility to spinal fractures.

Daily living and avoiding falls

During daily living, falls can happen at any age and at any time. I provide simple tips in order to decrease the risk of falls, especially if you have physical limitations due to advanced AS. Always wear a good pair of skid-resistant shoes. Avoid slippery surfaces and also avoid or get rid of loose rugs and carpets. Use stair railings and install grab bars in the shower, and some patients may need shower seats. Difficulty in using the toilet may require use of raised toilet seats and grab bars. Use of floor lighting or night lights is highly advised.

There are many devices to help perform daily tasks: walking canes, special chairs and desks, special shoes, and devices that assist in putting on socks or stockings and shoes, scratching the back, or applying soap and washing the back and lower legs, etc. Grabbers are very helpful for picking up items from the floor, especially if you also have severe hip joint involvement. Use a 3-wheeler or a 4-wheeler walker (the latter is safer to use) if you feel dizzy or are prone to falls. Car driving and other aspects of living are discussed in Chapter 21.

Spinal fractures

There are two types of vertebral spinal fractures: post-traumatic fractures and spontaneous compression fractures.

1. Post-traumatic spinal fracture

Patients with AS with a rigid osteoporotic spine have up to a 5-fold risk of post-traumatic spinal fracture and a 35% increased risk of vertebral compression fractures than the general population (Chapter 8, Figure 8.3). Approximately 80% of spinal fractures occur in the neck. Neurologic deficits are often subtle on initial presentation, resulting in the fracture being missed because of a low index of suspicion and poor visualization of lower cervical fractures on conventional X-rays. They occur more often following ground level falls in ~ 50% of patients versus ~ 7% in the general population. They may even occur following a relatively minor physical trauma, which may not even be recalled by some patients.

Any new-onset neck or back pain in a patient with AS, even in the absence of obvious physical trauma or after a seemingly trivial injury, should be evaluated for a spinal fracture and for any instability at the fracture site. Otherwise, it can unfortunately carry a risk of resultant paralysis of legs (paraplegia), or even of all four limbs (quadriplegia) in case of neck fracture. In case of a suspected spinal fracture, the patient may be better off lying on their side on the stretcher (rather than on their back), with a pillow under the head, when being transported to the hospital emergency room, so that the back and/or neck are immobilized in the patient's usual alignment. Excessive straightening into a "normal" position by extension of the ankylosed forward-stooping neck or thoracic spine during conventional immobilization or during X-ray and MRI procedures can result in new or worsen neurologic deficits. Neurological compromise can also occur during surgery to correct severe permanent forward stooping (kyphosis).

The spinal fracture usually occurs in the cervical spine, and MRI, CT, or bone scan results may be more helpful in confirming or excluding such spinal fracture than a neck X-ray. If you have a fused spine, it is wise for you to carry a suitable *personalized information card* that should state that your spine, including your neck, is fused because of AS, and that you are therefore much more prone to spinal fracture due to any fall or motor vehicle accident, even after a relatively trivial injury. The card should include your name, address, and phone number, a photograph (including a picture showing the spinal deformity), your blood group type, a list of medicines you are taking, any allergy history, and contact details of your doctor (Chapter 15 and Figure 15.1).

Patients with limited neck or spinal mobility should avoid manipulation of their back or neck by *chiropractors* and masseurs. Such treatments have sometimes inadvertently led to spinal fractures and neurological complications.

2. Spontaneous spinal vertebral compression fractures

Patients can also spontaneously get osteoporosis-related spinal compression (collapse) fractures or microfractures of one or more of their vertebral bodies. They more commonly involve midthoracic spine and can contribute to progressive spinal stooping, and ~ 75% of them are asymptomatic, detected only by reduction of the vertebral body height. They contribute to loss of body height and worsening of kyphosis of AS. In a person with osteoporosis in the general population unassociated with AS, usually an elderly woman, the hump occurs in the upper back (thoracic kyphosis), and the resultant stooped posture called "*dowager's hump*" may look superficially like AS.

Specialized bone density tests can detect osteoporosis before occurrence of a fracture and can also predict your chances of bone fracture in the future. Tests conducted at appropriate intervals can measure rate of bone loss and monitor treatment benefit. The best defense against developing osteoporosis in later life is to build strong bones during childhood and early adulthood. One needs to take a balanced diet rich in calcium and vitamin D and follow a healthy lifestyle. This requires performing regular weight-bearing exercise and avoidance of smoking. It has been estimated that an average woman acquires 98% of her total skeletal bone mass by about age 20 and she can lose up to 20% of her bone mass in the first 5 years after her menopause.

Asians and white women after age 65 in the general population are twice as likely as the African-American women to get fractures. Besides being female and the ethnicity, other predisposing (risk) factors include a family history of osteoporosis, having a small frame and very lean body, use of certain medications (e.g., corticosteroids), a diet low in calcium, excessive intake of alcohol, a sedentary (inactive lifestyle), and problems with keeping balance and tendency to falls. Elderly men can also, but less often, develop osteoporosis because of low testosterone levels.

23

Surgical treatment

 Key points

♦ General anesthesia can be a challenge for the anesthesiologist as they may have difficulty in passing a breathing tube down the trachea (windpipe) so that the airway can be maintained during general anesthesia for surgery.

♦ Do not assume that the surgical team is fully aware of all the limitations due to AS. You should discuss any concerns or apprehensions with the surgeon and also arrange a preoperative consultation with the anesthesiologist.

♦ Proper positioning for a surgical procedure is a shared responsibility of the surgeon, the anesthesiologist, and the rest of the operating team.

♦ Hip joint replacement is indicated in patients with advanced hip joint involvement and is a highly successful surgery.

♦ Heart complications, such as severe slowing of the heart or leaky heart valve may require placement of a cardiac (heart) pacemaker or valve replacement, respectively.

Anesthesia in people with AS

General anesthesia can be a challenge for the anesthesiologist as they may have difficulty in passing a breathing tube down the trachea (windpipe) so that the airway can be maintained during general anesthesia for surgery. This is a potential problem in anyone with a rigid spine, especially if you also have forwardly stooped neck or a reduced jaw-opening capacity. An instrument called a flexible *fiber optic laryngoscope* helps in putting the breathing tube down the trachea. However, someone with extreme neck deformity may require a *tracheostomy*. Patients with advanced AS who undergo any surgery requiring general anesthesia need good post-surgical care to avoid lung complications, which are more likely to occur due to their restricted chest wall movement.

Do not assume that healthcare providers are fully aware of all the limitations due to AS. You should discuss any concerns or apprehensions with the surgeon and arrange a preoperative consultation with the anesthesiologist. The anesthesiologist should examine you beforehand to find out your limitations and allay any concerns you may have. This should preferably be done in your hospital room, before you are taken to the operating room, and before you are given the anesthetic pre-medications that dim your alertness of mind. Proper positioning of the patient during surgery is a shared responsibility among the surgeon, the anesthesiologist, and the rest of the operating team.

Joint replacement (arthroplasty)

Hip joint involvement is seen in up to 20% of patients, especially among those with juvenile onset of the disease. Surgical replacement (arthroplasty) is indicated when patients have advanced hip joint involvement that is causing severe pain with impaired joint motion and functional impairment. It is a highly successful surgery in which part of pelvis (the cup-shaped socket) and thighbone (femur) that form the joint are replaced by an implant (prosthesis). It is called total hip arthroplasty (THA) in which the socket is replaced by durable plastic cup surrounded by metal shell, and the head and part of the neck of the femur is replaced by a metal ball attached to a metal stem that is inserted into the top of the femur (Figure 23.1). Minimally invasive total hip arthroplasty is a newer technique that needs smaller incisions than traditional surgery. The patient experiences less pain and recovers more quickly, with a resultant shorter stay in the hospital.

Hip arthroplasty gives very good result and, to a large extent, prevents partial or total disability from severe hip disease. However, it requires physical therapy for 6–8 weeks after discharge from the hospital. In general, the prosthesis remains functional for up to 20 years, and in some patients, it can last even longer. A hip revision surgery may be needed when it gets worn out or becomes loose.

Similarly, the involvement of the other joints, especially the knees, may require joint replacement in advanced cases. People who are about to undergo elective joint replacement surgeries should be in good general and dental health. If it is difficult to intubate for general anesthesia, for example due to severe forward stooping of the neck, *epidural* spinal anesthesia is an alternative. Lumbar spinal anesthesia may not be possible because of inability to perform lumbar puncture in patients with a totally fused lumbar spine.

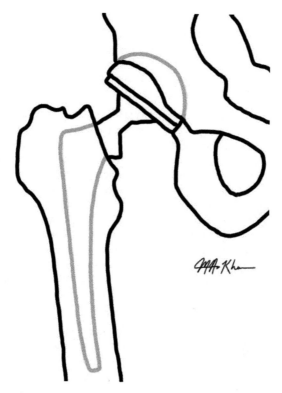

Figure 23.1 Schematic drawing showing a total arthroplasty of right hip joint.

Infection can be a serious complication of arthroplasties, but with advances in the use of antibiotics and other technical aspects, the occurrence of infections has been markedly reduced in recent years. Bacteria can travel through the blood and infect a total joint implant, both in the early postoperative period and for some years following implantation; however the most critical period is the first 2 years after joint replacement. Dental and endoscopic procedures can cause temporary circulation of bacteria in the blood, so people with artificial joints undergoing these procedures may need prophylactic antibiotics to minimize the risk of infection affecting the replaced joint.

Other surgical procedures

Spinal surgery may be needed for stabilization of spinal fracture. Severe spinal forward curvature (kyphosis) used to occur in some people with severe

AS, but its occurrence should now be very uncommon if the disease is diagnosed at an early stage and treated appropriately. Such a severe kyphosis can be surgically corrected for someone so bent that they cannot look straight ahead. However, such a surgery carries a relatively high risk of paraplegia and high morbidity among very elderly patients. This aspect should be clearly discussed with the patient and carefully weighed against benefit.

Heart complications, such as leaky heart valve or severe slowing of the heartbeat, may require valve replacement or the placement of a cardiac (heart) pacemaker, respectively. Transcatheter aortic valve replacement (TAVR) is a minimally invasive procedure to replace a narrowed aortic valve that fails to open properly (aortic valve stenosis). It is the aortic valve incompetence (leaky aortic valve) that is associated with AS, whereas aortic valve stenosis is associated with progressive calcium deposition in the aortic valve with advancing age, and it is unrelated to AS. I underwent TAVR procedure in June 2022 for my calcific aortic stenosis that is unrelated to my AS. I walked into the hospital using my three-wheeled walker at 7:30 am and walked out of the hospital at 7:30 pm the same day with a new aortic valve without any stitches on my body. A year earlier I had placement of a cardiac pacemaker (installed under the skin on my upper chest wall) for severe slowing of my heartbeat that was related to my living with AS for 66 years.

Scarring (fibrosis) and cavity (cyst) formation in the upper part (apex) of the lung are now very rare but still not easy to manage and surgical removal of diseased tissue may sometimes be required.

24

Non-traditional (complementary or alternative) therapy

➔ Key points

◆ Unlike conventional medicines, nutritional supplements and herbal preparations are not regulated by agencies such as the FDA.

◆ People are therefore using many of these substances without any certainty about their precise composition, strength, and dose, and without scientifically valid proof of their safety or effectiveness.

◆ Some practitioners providing complementary medicine do not need to have a license or other proof of their competency to prescribe such remedies or procedures.

◆ This chapter provides detailed discussion of the various non-traditional (complementary or alternative) remedies and procedures that have lately become more popular, including the various diets, probiotics, and nutritional or dietary supplements that also fall in the category of alternative approaches to disease management. Tai Chi and Yoga are discussed on page 99.

◆ The efficacy and safety of acupuncture as a treatment of AS is not supported by the published data.

◆ Proper use of the Internet to obtain medical information is discussed (and also in Chapter 13).

Ankylosing Spondylitis and Axial Spondyloarthritis, Second Edition. Muhammad Asim Khan, Oxford University Press.
© Oxford University Press 2023. DOI: 10.1093/oso/9780198864158.003.0024

Introduction

Non-traditional therapies (complementary and alternative or folk remedies) for arthritis have lately become more popular, and the US population spends lot of money on these unproven treatments. People use such treatments for many reasons, such as lack of adequate relief with many conventional arthritis medicines or their untoward effects. Another reason is that many conventional medical and surgical treatments are quite costly. Moreover, arthritis treatment attracts charlatans peddling "miracle cures."

These therapies that include traditional Chinese medicine (such as acupuncture), massage therapy, homeopathy, naturopathic remedies, nutritional supplements and multivitamins, herbal preparations, and others. Unlike conventional use of remedies (as surgery or drugs or other measures that have proved of value in treatment of disease (allopathy)), non-traditional therapies are not regulated by agencies such as the FDA. People are therefore using many of these remedies without any certainty about their precise strength, composition, and dose, and without scientifically valid proof of their safety or effectiveness. Their use is based on anecdotal evidence, mostly from individuals who report their own successful use of the treatment. Scientific methods should be applied to establish the validity of the anecdotal evidence. Moreover, some practitioners providing complementary medicine do not need to have a license or other proof of their competency to prescribe such remedies or procedures.

Sometimes people benefit from non-traditional remedies because of the *placebo effect* (due to patient's belief in that treatment), and on other occasions they may experience coincidental "cure" because many rheumatic diseases can have cyclical spontaneous disease flare-ups and remissions. It is tempting to credit relief of symptoms to the complementary medicine that, just by chance, was started when the disease was beginning to go into remission, even though the medicine may really have had no effect on the disease.

It is important to emphasize that there is no rigorous scientific evidence to support the use of such therapies by people with AS. There are many quacks preying on the pain and suffering of vulnerable or desperate people. These quacks may promote or promise questionable and sometimes outright dangerous treatments as "cures" and may even harm people, not only financially but also medically, by keeping them away from effective therapies.

The National Center for Complementary and Integrative Health

The National Center for Complementary and Integrative Health (<http://www.nccih.nih.gov>) recommends that people should take the following steps before trying any complementary therapy.

Always let your doctor know if you plan to or are already taking any complementary therapy because some therapies may potentially interact with the medicines that you may be currently taking as prescribed by your doctor or affect other illnesses that you may have.

Ask the healthcare provider or the complementary therapy practitioner about the expected beneficial results, risks, costs, and length of treatment. Some forms of them may be expensive because they are not usually covered by health insurance.

Check the credentials of the practitioner. Research the expertise of the practitioner or salesperson associated with a given treatment. Check with your local or state business bureau if you are going to buy a product from a business. Testimonials of other people with arthritis who have tried a complementary or alternative treatment cannot prove how safe or effective the treatment will be for others. Obtain objective scientific information about it at a library or through reliable Internet sources.

Diets, probiotics, and prebiotics

Diet is also often considered an "alternative" approach to disease management. There is yet no special diet or a specific food that can prevent AS/axSpA or alleviate its severity. But patients claiming benefit from certain dietary changes may be describing something other than a placebo effect.

Elimination diets that require you to stop eating certain foods have been tried without any clear benefit in the management of AS. One investigator has been touting possible beneficial effect of a *low-starch diet*. It involves a reduced intake of bread, potatoes, cakes, and pasta. However, this diet has not been scientifically evaluated and there has been no independent scientifically valid confirmation of its overall benefit. It is therefore not recommended.

Probiotics are yeast- and certain human-derived live bacteria that contribute to digestive health. Yogurt and kefir are widely regarded as the best sources of probiotics; they are both dairy products made from fermented milk. Consumption of yogurt can help some patient in reducing abdominal symptoms and diarrhea caused by antibiotics use, IBD, infectious diarrhea (caused by viruses, bacteria, or parasites), and irritable bowel syndrome (IBS). Other types of probiotics include salted and fermented vegetables, such as sauerkraut, kimchi, Japanese natto, and Indonesian tempeh (or tempe), but they are not suitable for people on dietary salt restriction because of their very high salt content.

Prebiotics are a component of some foods that the body cannot digest. The indigestible fibers (or roughage) provide no calories and can prevent constipation. However, they serve as food for bacteria and other beneficial microbes in the gut and increase their variety. Since they occur naturally in many foods, there is no need to take prebiotic supplements. There is currently no evidence that taking prebiotics and probiotics together is harmful. However, research on potential side effects of probiotics and prebiotics requires further investigation. Before you try to incorporate them into your diet, you need to speak with a dietitian or knowledgeable healthcare practitioner first. People who have chronic diseases or serious illnesses should avoid probiotic or prebiotic supplements without a doctor's advice.

Intermittent fasting is a dietary intervention that focuses on timing when a person can eat within a day or within a week. The two prominent patterns are "alternate day fasting" and "time-restricted eating." The latter pattern involves anywhere between 16 and 20 hours daily fast with 4–8 hours feeding time. These eating patterns improve many health indices, even without reduction of total calorie intake, such as reduction in abdominal fat, improvement in physical endurance, glucose metabolism, and blood pressure control. They have also shown potential benefit in slowing down Alzheimer's and Parkinson's diseases.

Nutritional supplements

Nutritional or dietary supplements, as their name suggests, are being used to supplement the diet, but they are largely unregulated. They can contain vitamins C, E, and A, omega-3 fatty acids glucosamine and chondroitin sulfate, and S-Adenosylmethionine (SAM-e, pronounced "Sam-ee"), a compound that occurs naturally in all human tissues and has been used in Europe for years as a medication for arthritis and depression, and other ingredients. One should not take nutritional supplements just because friends or family members are taking them, and it is wise to first consult your physician or dietician. A Canadian survey of people with osteoarthritis found that many of them had used a variety of complementary therapies, but only 30% of them had discussed this with their doctors.

There are circumstances where one may benefit from use of certain vitamins. For example, vitamin D supplement is needed for people with poor dietary intake and low vitamin D level, or those with inadequate sun exposure because they stay indoors, those who, for various reasons, wear clothing that limits their sun exposure; or if they suffer from conditions that limit fat absorption because vitamin D is a fat-soluble vitamin. Eggs, mushrooms, and oily fish such as salmon are good dietary sources of vitamin D. Over-supplementation can be dangerous because vitamin D, like other fat-soluble vitamins A, E, and K, is stored in the body for a long period and overdosage can result in toxicity. The water-soluble vitamins B and C if taken in excess are quickly excreted in the urine.

It is wise to treat all supplements, not just pills, as drugs that can be dangerous for people taking certain prescription medications. Vitamin E supplement can increase the risk of bleeding in people taking anticoagulant or anti-platelet medicines, such as warfarin. Vitamin K, on the other hand, can promote clotting by interacting with warfarin. Some studies have suggested that tobacco smokers who take high doses of beta-carotene vitamin B-complex supplements have a higher risk of lung cancer.

Traditional Chinese medicine

The ancient *traditional Chinese system of medicine* (TCM) includes herbal and nutritional supplements, meditation, acupuncture, and restorative physical exercises and massage.

Herbs are the basis for many traditional medicines, such as aspirin, morphine, and digitalis, and practitioners of some complementary therapies believe that certain herbs have anti-inflammatory effects. Many of the herbal therapies that are now used in complementary or alternative medicine were used by the mainstream medical profession up until the early part of the twentieth century in the Western world. Many of them are still considered mainstream medicine in some poorer regions of the world that lack modern healthcare and its effective therapies. Some herbs contain powerful and potentially toxic substances that can interfere with other medications that you may be taking, so you should talk to your doctor before taking any herbal preparation.

The regular practice of *meditation* helps you to enter a deeply restful and relaxed state, with a reduction in the body's stress response, slowing of brain waves and heartbeat, and decrease in muscle tension. *Tai Chi* is a traditional Chinese mind–body relaxation exercise system, discussed in Chapter 8.

Acupuncture

Acupuncture is based on the Chinese concept of balanced Qi (pronounced "chee"), or vital energy, that flows throughout the body via 12 main and 8 secondary pathways (called meridians), accessed through the more than 2,000 acupuncture points on the human body. It is one of the oldest medical procedures in the world, originating in China more than 2,000 years ago. It is believed to remove the imbalances of Yin (negative energy and forces in the universe and human body) and Yang (positive energy). This brings the body into balance, keeps the normal flow of the vital energy Qi unblocked, and restores health to the mind and body.

Acupuncture became widely known in the US in 1971 when *New York Times* reporter James Reston wrote about how doctors in China eased his abdominal pain by puncturing the skin with hair-thin needles at particular locations. Although the mechanism of action is unclear, stimulation of acupuncture points may lead to release by the brain and spinal cord (via the endorphin system) of opium-like molecules (neurotransmitters and neurohormones), that help to modulate pain. But the same can happen also after vigorous exercise.

Acupuncture could work for some conditions due to its placebo effect. It has been shown that a real drug, naloxone (which inhibits endorphin-producing cells in the brain), can reverse pain relief obtained by placebo (sham) painkiller; this indicates that in some cases placebo works via the endorphin system. The Chinese claim that acupuncture can also lead to biochemical changes that may stimulate healing and promote general well-being.

The WHO, which is the health branch of the United Nations, lists more than 40 conditions for which acupuncture is used, including non-specific back and neck pain, and arthritis. This is based on mostly anecdotal evidence, mostly from people who report their own successful use of the treatment. The efficacy safety of acupuncture as a treatment of AS is not supported by the published data. Scientific studies are under way to establish the validity of the anecdotal evidence of the potential benefit of acupuncture in some forms of arthritis.

Other therapies

Chiropractic treatment: As mentioned in Chapter 22, patients with AS/axSpA or anyone with limited neck or spinal mobility should avoid manipulation of their neck and/or their back by *chiropractors* and masseurs because such treatments have sometimes inadvertently led to spinal fractures and neurological complications.

Hypnosis has been used to promote relaxation and help a person cope better with pain. Another proposed way of achieving a restful and relaxed state is by *guided imagery*, which involves creating a vivid and pleasant mental picture. For example, you might see yourself sitting on a beach on a warm day, looking at the waves and hearing them pounding on the shore.

Biofeedback is a related method that involves using various machines that monitor one's body temperature, heart rate, breathing patterns, and other bodily functions, and provide feedback that helps you to learn how to produce these effects and a feeling of relaxation voluntarily, without the need for machine monitors.

Holistic medicine deals with an integrated comprehensive overview of a physical, mental, emotional, and spiritual being; practitioners may suggest therapies based on the whole person, including spiritual and mental aspects, not just the specific part of the body being treated. They may advise changes in diet, lifestyle, and physical activity to help treat your condition.

TENS (transcutaneous electrical nerve stimulation) is a technique that requires placing electrodes on the skin to convey an electric current to nerve cells. It is of no value for people with AS.

Ayurveda, the traditional Indian system of medicine, is also not effective in AS.

Homeopathy uses extremely diluted preparations of natural substances, such as plants and minerals, and scientists are skeptical about its effectiveness. A study of the homeopathic treatment with "Formica ruta" concluded that it is not effective in AS.

Bee and snake venom are used by some alternative practitioners who claim that bee venom relieves the symptoms of rheumatoid arthritis because it contains certain enzymes and stimulates the body to produce more corticosteroids. This treatment is potentially dangerous for about 10% of the population who have mild, severe, or even fatal allergic reactions to insect venom. Snake venom is toxic and there is little scientific support for its use in treating arthritis.

Dimethyl sulfoxide (DMSO) is an industrial solvent like turpentine, and the industrial-grade DMSO sold in hardware stores may contain harmful contaminants. Some people believe that DMSO or its breakdown product *methyl sulfonyl methane* (MSM) can relieve pain and reduce swelling when rubbed on the skin, but rheumatologists do not recommend this unproven treatment.

The wearing of *copper bracelets*, according to folk lore, allows trace amounts of copper to be absorbed through the skin and neutralize toxic molecules called free radicals that can otherwise damage tissues. There is no scientific basis for their medical benefit but appear to be harmless and may have some placebo effect. Same is true for the use of *magnets*. *Aromatherapy* (where patients are asked to inhale oils derived from plant extracts and resins, or these substances are massaged into their skin) also has no place in managing AS.

Radiation (X-ray) treatment of the spine has no role in the modern management of AS. It can result in cancer (read Case 2, Chapter 26). Use of combined low-dose radon/hyperthermia "baths" in mines are still used in some German-speaking countries but are not advised.

What is medical cannabis (medical marijuana)?

Cannabis plant is the source of marijuana (herbal cannabis) refers to the dried buds and leaves from two strains of *Cannabis* plant (*c. indica* and *c. sativa*). Hashish refers to resin or compressed resin glands from the buds of the plant. People use cannabis products by inhalation of the smoke or by eating or mixing it with drinks.

Medical cannabis specifically refers to its use for medicinal purposes, and it contains specific amounts of molecules called tetrahydrocannabinol (THC) and cannabidiol (CBD). THC has a psychoactive (mind-altering) property, and its effects are characterized by impairment of psychomotor and cognitive performance, as well as a range of physical effects that include dry mouth and rapid heartbeat. CBD does not produce the effects that are typically seen with THC and is generally well tolerated with a very low likelihood of dependence (addiction). The primary source of CBD is hemp (a closely related plant and its stalks have been used for its fiber since ancient times) because it contains a very low (less than 0.3%) concentration of THC.

Use of CBD is not approved or regulated by the FDA in the US, but people are using it to help manage symptoms like sleep disturbance, fatigue, and chronic pain. You should discuss with your physician prior to its use because it may interact with some of your other medications, most notably sedatives, sleeping tablets, pain medications, certain high blood pressure medications (antihypertensives), and anticoagulants ("blood thinners").

CBD is consumed as cream, pills, oil, or inhaled sprays; the most reliable and safest way is to use the oil as drops under the tongue. There is no standard regulation that ensures that the product packaging reflects its contents. Therefore, there may be no assurance that you are getting what you are paying for. You may need to check if it has a Certificate of Analysis (COA) that shows the quantity of the various ingredients.

To date, research and clinical trials of herbal cannabis are very limited and conflicting results have been reported. The strongest scientific evidence for CBD effectiveness is in treating certain forms of severe childhood epilepsy which may not respond to anti-seizure medications. The WHO issued a detail report on the pharmacology, safety, and effectiveness of CBD in November 2017 (<https://www.who.int/medicines/access/controlled-substances/5.2_CBD.pdf>).

Lastly, it is very important for you to know that CBD use will cause you to have a positive urine drug screening test for marijuana, and if your job requires drug screening, this may cause problems.

Cautionary note regarding use of the Internet

Doctors should encourage their patients to be well informed about their disease; such patients will comply better with treatment and also better understand the rationale for their treatment. Much useful information can be obtained from the Internet, as discussed in detail in Chapter 13. You can find objective scientific information from reliable sources, such as the National Institutes of Health (NIH) and MedlinePlus at <http://www.nlm.nih.gov/medlineplus>. Appendix 1 gives contact details for some very reputable AS patient organizations, which are also a useful source of information. The Internet-savvy patients' ability to obtain relevant information need not adversely impact their patient/physician relationship if openly discussed with their health care providers. However, be aware that there is a huge amount of misinformation out there that can be potentially harmful. You should be very careful and "not believe everything that washes ashore while you are surfing the Net."

25

Disease course and effect on life span

 Key points

- The course of the disease is highly variable, and the spine does not always fuse completely as the disease may stay limited to the SI joints and the lower lumbar spine in some patients. Spinal structural damage seems to progress most rapidly when patients are 30–39 years of age.

- In women, the spine fusion (ankylosis) tends to progress more slowly, and neck pain, anterior chest wall pain and tenderness (costochondritis), and limb joint involvement may be the main manifestations.

- There is no cure yet for AS, but most patients can be very well managed with increasingly more effective medications and life-long programs of regular physical exercises.

- In general, most patients do well and continue to live normal and productive lives, although some may have to modify their lifestyle or their work environment.

- There is a need for early disease detection, more effective anti-inflammatory treatment with b-DMARDs (biologics) and ts-DMARDs, as well as prevention and management and of comorbid conditions.

Disease course

The course of the disease is highly variable, and most patients do well and continue to live normal and productive lives, although some may have to modify their lifestyle or their work environment. Some patients may only have a series of mild aches and pains, coming and going for months. Others have more chronic back pain that leads to varying degree of spinal stiffness and gradually decreasing spinal mobility, leading to worsening physical function.

As discussed in Chapter 1, the disease symptoms and severity not only vary from one person to another but also between males and females. In general, there is a gradual progression of the disease over the years, but slower and relatively incomplete progression of spinal fusion among woman may mean that it takes longer for their pain to decrease (that results from complete spinal ankylosis).

The patients with slow disease progression can be minimally symptomatic or almost pain-free for long periods of time, and in others the disease may not progress to complete spinal ankylosis because the inflammation may ease off before this can happen, especially with effective management and patient's full compliance. For some patients, the first symptoms may not be back pain but painful girdle (hip and shoulder) or limb joints, or heel pain. In some such cases it may be difficult to distinguish the disease from some other rheumatic diseases before the emergence of typical back symptoms.

Spinal structural damage in AS seems to progress most rapidly when patients are 30–39 years of age. CRP elevation at baseline; history of smoking, history of acute anterior uveitis, presence of syndesmophytes (bony bridging of vertebra) at baseline, and higher grades of sacroiliitis at baseline are independent risk factors for severe disease. Others include being male, HLA-B27-positive, obese, and having a history of or persistent peripheral joint involvement.

In people with the progressive form of the disease, as the spinal ankylosis gradually worsens, the inflammatory back pain regresses because inflammation gets replaced by a healing process that involves new bone formation. This is sometimes referred to as "burning out" of the disease. However, some occasional features of the disease such as episodic eye inflammation (acute anterior uveitis) and heel pain may continue to occur, suggesting that the disease may not have gone into complete remission. Some may seek medical attention for development of psoriasis or for symptoms of frequency and urgency of bowel movement, bloating, or abdominal pain due to IBD.

Life span

Previous reports had reported shortening of life span, possibly resulting from cardiovascular (heart attack and stroke) and pulmonary diseases that are compounded by excessive smoking, spinal fractures due to fall or other form of physical trauma, alcoholism-related injury, gastrointestinal bleeding, miscellaneous conditions (such as associated IBD and psoriasis, amyloidosis, and cancer or lymphoma resulting from radiation treatment that was in use till

1950s). These older studies included patients whose disease was severe enough to impel them to seek medical care and get diagnosed at a time when AS was considered to be a rare disease and no effective treatments were available.

Recent studies still show a somewhat shorter survival of people with AS than the general population, and it is significantly associated with a lower level of education and socio-economic status, smoking, diabetes, infections, heart and lung diseases, malignancy, previous hip replacement surgery, spinal fracture, work disability, duration and intensity of inflammation, delayed diagnosis, and not using any affective therapy. It is very likely that the survival of patients with milder disease, who form a majority of patients with axSpA that encompasses AS and nr-axSpA, and receiving more effective therapies will have a normal life-span when compared with the general population.

There is still a need for earlier disease detection and more effective drug treatment (with NSAIDs/bDMARDs/ts-DMARD), life-long physical exercises, prevention of spinal fracture, as well as better management and prevention of comorbid conditions, such as unhealthy lifestyle (smoking, excessive alcohol use, obesity), diabetes, hypertension, high cholesterol, and heart and lung diseases. Male patients more often tend to be overweight or obese, and more frequently have unhealthy alcohol intake.

26

Brief illustrative case histories

Case 1

Adam, a 26-year-old college student, presented with chronic back pain. He had been quite well up until 18 months ago, when he started having low back pain and stiffness. He initially felt the pain in his buttocks area for a few months, and then it progressed to involve his lower back as well, It was associated with back stiffness that was worsened by prolonged sitting, and at night and on waking up in the morning.

His stated that his back symptoms are worse when he first wakes up gets out of bed in the morning, but they start easing up after an hour, or earlier with physical activity or exercise, and after a hot shower. In the last 3 months, Adam has noticed pain and tenderness in his anterior (front) chest well (rib cage) around his breastbone that is accentuated on coughing or sneezing. He has no history of chronic diarrhea, skin disease, eye inflammation, or injury to his back. His father was killed in a car accident at the age of 30, and he is the only child. His paternal uncle has had a stiff back and neck for many years.

On physical examination, Adam was found to have tenderness over his SI joints, the lumbar spine, anterior chest wall (costochondritis), tenderness over his right jaw joint (temporo-mandibular joint, or TMJ for short), as well as limitation of motion of his lumbar spine. His chest expansion on full inspiration was normal but painful, and the rest of his physical examination was normal. Because these clinical findings indicated a strong probability of AS, an X-ray of his pelvis was ordered. The presence of bilateral sacroiliitis on the X-ray confirmed the diagnosis of AS.

He was educated about his illness and its appropriate management, including a life-long exercise program, appropriate counseling, and was also given a pamphlet about his illness. He is very computer savvy and was also given the Internet

Ankylosing Spondylitis and Axial Spondyloarthritis, Second Edition. Muhammad Asim Khan, Oxford University Press.
© Oxford University Press 2023. DOI: 10.1093/oso/9780198864158.003.0026

addresses of reputable patient self-help societies and organizations. He was prescribed an NSAID to be taken with meals but it was changed to another at 2 weeks because of lack of adequate response. At 1 month follow-up he showed minimal improvement. After performing further screening tests and discussion with him about the benefits and potential risk of untoward effects of other treatment options, he was started on a TNF inhibitor with subsequent good response.

Case 2

This case-history is excerpted and updated from the actual life story of a remarkable Swiss patient that I published in 2016 (Khan MA. "Accomplishments of Heinz Baumberger PhD: A remarkable patient with ankylosing spondylitis for 72 years" *Clin Rheumatol.* 2016;35(6):1637–41). He passed away in September 2020, 3 months short of his 90th birthday, having lived a remarkably productive life with severe form of AS for 78 years.

His symptoms began at age 12 and he had already developed a stiff back by the time he reached high school and was unable to join in school gymnastics or play with his friends or ski. His disease was finally diagnosed 10 years later in 1953 at age 22. He was treated with a 3-week course of spinal radiation that was being used at that time to provide some benefit for patients with severe disease. He was called up for military training service but was not accepted because of his AS.

By the time he married in 1957, his back pain and stiffness had become so severe that he needed his wife's help in washing, dressing, and even getting into and out of bed. By the early 1960s he had lost mobility of whole of his spine, including his neck. During his job as a schoolteacher, he started taking classes learning biology at a university in his spare time, but this double burden over those years had sapped his health almost to a breaking point, and his wife and two daughters had been through very hard times.

He received a second 3-week course of spinal radiation in 1962 that brought a certain degree of relief, but it greatly undermined his general health. He was prescribed NSAIDs that had become available then, and he found them to be helpful, but the recommended physical therapy made matters worse. Only gradually did he overcome his resistance to physical therapy, and together with his daily use of NSAIDs he was finally able to sleep better after more than 15 years of not having had a proper night's sleep. From that time onwards, he also regularly went every year for 4 weeks of intensive physical therapy along with warm water hydrotherapy (spa) and swimming. The pain in his back, chest, and neck finally abated after 35 years and he started enjoying this new lease of life.

He had suffered from "primary AS," without any associated psoriasis or IBD, and none of his immediate family members suffered from AS or these associated diseases. He did possess HLA-B27 and had many severe episodes of inflammation of his eyes (acute anterior uveitis).

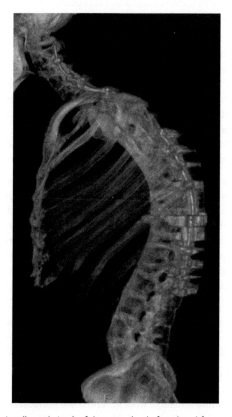

Figure 26.1 Imaging (lateral view) of the completely fused and forwardly stooped (kyphotic) spine of the second patient after more than 75 years of the disease. It also shows the metallic hardware that was needed to fix his spinal fractures sustained on 3 separate occasions. Notice the "squaring" and bone thinning (osteoporosis) of the fused lumbar vertebrae and conversion of the inter-vertebral discs into bone. However, it is remarkable that the holes through which the lumbar nerve come out at the back of the lumbar vertebrae are intact

Reproduced with permission from Baumberger H, Giovanni ME, Khan MA. Description of «Panoramic Field» for Assessment of Impaired Ability of Ankylosing Spondylitis Patients to Fully See Their Surroundings Despite Having Normal Field of Vision. *Rheuma Schweiz Fachzeitschrift*. 2019, 6:30–34.

He had sustained his spinal fractures (Figure 26.1) from falls on three different occasions. His last fracture was of his neck that happened a couple of days after his discharge from a hospital following treatment of severe infection with abscesses and lack of healing after an excision of six skin cancers (basal cell carcinomas) on his back that were attributed to his two courses of spinal radiation many decades ago, a well-documented late complication of such treatment that is not used anymore.

It was only in 1971 that he first met another person with AS, and it was a great help to him to subsequently seek out and meet other patients to hear their experiences. As a result of such conversations, he and three other patients formed a patient support group in 1977 and called it the "Schweizerische Vereinigung Morbus Bechterew" (SVMB for short; Swiss Ankylosing Spondylitis Society). In German speaking countries AS is quite often called Morbus Bechterew. He subsequently found out that theirs was the second such AS patient support group in the world; the first being the National Ankylosing Spondylitis Society (NASS) in England, now renamed National Axial Spondyloarthritis Society.

He also took upon himself to gain extensive knowledge about AS and, with his rheumatologist, co-authored an excellent and well-illustrated book on AS (Paul Schmied and Heinz Baumberger, Morbus Bechterew: der entzündliche Wirbelsäulen-Rheumatismus. Published by Urban and Fischer, Munich. 2002. ISBN: 3437457063, 9783437457067). For patients and their family members, and allied health professionals in German language. His self-gained knowledge about the occurrence of spinal fractures in AS and how medical emergency services should handle patients with presumed spinal fractures was very instrumental in preventing spinal cord damage after each of his three spinal fractures.

He made more than 45 trips abroad, lecturing and participating in various scientific meetings and congresses in Europe, Asia, and the Americas in his zeal to spread the idea of self-help organizations for patients with AS.

I had known and collaborated with him since 1983, and on my last communication with him, 10 days before he passed away, he was delighted to know that all five of our scientific abstracts were accepted for presentation at the annual meeting of the American College of Rheumatology. They were the result of a 35-years-long Swiss family study of AS patients that could not have been performed without his help and participation. The first manuscript resulting from that study was published posthumously in March 2022 (van der Linden SM, Khan MA, Li Z, et al. "Factors predicting axial spondyloarthritis among first-degree relatives of probands with ankylosing spondylitis. A family study spanning 35 years" *Ann Rheum Dis.* 2022 March. <http://dx.doi.org/10.1136/annrheumdis-2021-222083>).

Appendix 1

Patient support groups and other helpful organizations

ACR (American College of Rheumatology) <http://www.rheumatology.org> is a US professional membership organization founded in 1934. It also provides information for patients and caregivers.

APLAR (Asia and Pacific League Against Rheumatism) <http://www.aplar.org>.

Arthritis Foundation <http://arthritis.org> is the largest nonprofit advocacy group focused on finding a cure and championing the fight against arthritis in the United States.

Arthritis Society <http://arthritis.ca> is a similar nonprofit advocacy group in Canada focused on finding a cure and championing the fight against arthritis. Another society is the **AAC** (Arthritis Alliance of Canada) at <http://www.arthritisalliance,ca>.

ASIF (Axial Spondyloarthritis International Federation) <http://www.asif.info/en> was established in 1988 to increase public awareness of AS/axSpA, and to disseminate knowledge of the disease around the world. It currently has 51 patient organization members from 44 countries around the world. Its website lists and web links for many patients support and advocacy groups, societies, and organizations throughout the globe, but only 3 of them are listed here:

1. **NASS** (National Axial Spondyloarthritis Society) <http:/www.nass.co.uk> is the first such patient advocacy and support society established in the United Kingdom in 1976.

2. **SVMB** (Schweizerische Vereinigung Morbus Bechterew) <http://www.bechterew.ch> is the second oldest patient advocacy and support society that was established in Switzerland in 1977. Its name can be translated in English to Swiss Ankylosing Spondylitis Society

3. SAA (Spondylitis Association of America) <http://www.spondylitis.org> is the most important and largest patient advocacy and support organization in the United States.

ASAS <http://www.asas-group.org>, **SPARTAN** <http://www.spartangroup.org>, and **GRAPPA** <http:www.grappanetwork.org> are the 3 members-only networks of healthcare professionals dedicated to research and education in AS and the related forms of SpA.

CDC (Centers for Disease Control and Prevention) <http://www.cdc.gov> is the US health protection agency whose goal is to help save lives and protect people from health, safety, and security threats.

EMA (Europeans Medicines Agency) <http://www.ema.europa.eu> is responsible for the scientific evaluation, supervision, and safety monitoring of medicines developed by pharmaceutical companies for use in the European Union.

EULAR (European Alliance of Associations for Rheumatology) <http://www.eular.org> has just published recommendations for self-management in people with types of inflammatory arthritis. The original publication can be downloaded free from their website.

FDA (Food and Drug Administration) <http://www.fda.gov> is responsible for protecting the public health in the United States by ensuring the safety, efficacy, and security of human and veterinary drugs, biological products, etc.

ILAR (International League of Associations for Rheumatology) <http://www.ilar.org> comprises partner professional membership organizations from around the world that are committed to improving the care of patients with rheumatic diseases and advancing the rheumatology subspecialty. It includes ACR, EULAR, PANLAR, APLAR, and AFLAR.

MedlinePlus <http://www.medlineplus.gov/healthtopics.html> is an online and very reliable health information source for patients and their families and friends.

NCCIH (National Center for Complementary and Integrative Health) <http://www.nccih.nih.gov> is a part of the NIH that provides the most authentic information about complementary and alternative remedies and procedures.

NHS (National Health Service) <http://www.nhs.uk> is the biggest government-funded health-related website in Britain that provides very useful information.

NICE (National Institute for Health and Clinical Excellence) <http://www.nice.org.uk> of the UK's National Health Service publishes guidelines for the use of health technologies, clinical practice, health promotion and ill-health avoidance, and social care services.

NIH (National Institute of Health) <http://www.nih.gov> is a part of the US government Department of Health and Human Services. It is the world's foremost and largest medical research agency, and its many websites provide the latest and most useful health-related and research information.

NLM (National Library of Medicine) <http://www.nlm.nih.gov> is the world's largest medical library and is a part of the NIH.

PANLAR (Pan-American League Against Rheumatism) <http://www.pan lar.org>.

WHO (World Health Organization) <http://www.who.org> works with 194 member states with the aim to achieve better health for everyone, everywhere in the world.

HLAB27.com is a free website **<http://www.HLAB27.com>** by the author for patients and their relatives, the general public, and for students, physicians, and allied health professionals on the topics of AS/axSpA and HLA-B27, and it also provides some of the authors publication.

Appendix 2

Glossary

Achilles tendinitis inflammation of the Achilles tendon, causing swelling and tenderness at the lower end of the calf where it inserts into the heel bone

ACR American College of Rheumatology

acupuncture an ancient medical procedure that originated in China more than 2,000 years ago. It is based on the theoretical concept of balanced Qi (pronounced 'chee') or vital energy that flows throughout the body via certain pathways that are accessed by puncturing the skin with hair-thin needles at particular locations called **acupuncture points**. Stimulation of acupuncture points is believed to stimulate the brain and spinal cord to release chemicals that change the experience of pain or cause biochemical changes that may stimulate healing and promote general well-being. See also **alternative and complementary remedies, traditional Chinese medicine**

acute anterior uveitis indicates inflammation of the anterior parts of the eye that comprises iris and ciliary body; it is sometimes also called acute iritis or acute uveitis

allele alternate forms of a gene at a distinct location (locus) on a chromosome

alternative and complementary remedies these include holistic medicine, folk remedies, and alternative therapies (herbal medications or extracts, homeopathy, Ayurvedics, and traditional Chinese medicine (TCM)). These complementary and alternative treatments are mostly based on anecdotal evidence, primarily from individuals who report their own successful use of the treatment. One needs to apply scientific methods to establish the validity of the anecdotal evidence

amino acids small organic molecules which are the building blocks of peptides and proteins

amyloid a proteinaceous fibrillar material deposited in various tissues and organs, sometimes secondary to a chronic inflammatory disease

analgesia pain relief, e.g., by such drugs as paracetamol, **NSAIDs** or narcotics. These pain-relieving drugs are called **analgesics** (see NSAIDs)

ankylosing hyperostosis also called **Forestier's disease** or **diffuse idiopathic skeletal hyperostosis** (DISH). It causes excessive new bone formation along the spine and other sites (such as entheses), can result in stiff spine that may be confused with AS

ankylosing spondylitis (AS) an inflammatory arthritic disorder, primarily of the axial skeleton (sacroiliac joints and spine) but can affect hip and shoulder joints and infrequently the peripheral joints. It causes chronic back pain and leads to stiffness of the spine. Most of the affected individuals have the HLA-B27 gene

ankylosis fusion, which may be fibrous, or bony (as in AS)

annulus fibrosus the tough outer fibrous layer of the intervertebral disc

anterior chest wall pain is usually the result of arthritis involving the attachment of the collar bones (clavicles) and the ribs to the breastbone comprising manubrium and sternum. Also see **costochondritis**

antibodies proteins produced by white blood cells (plasma cells and B lymphocytes) that confer immunity

antigen a substance that causes the body's immune system to produce antibodies that try to eliminate it because the body sees the antigen as foreign or harmful substance (e.g., from invading viruses or bacteria)

antigen-presenting cell a cell that ingests and processes foreign substance (e.g., from invading viruses or bacteria) and displays the resulting antigen fragments (small peptides) on its surface to activate those T cells that respond specifically to that antigen

aortitis inflammation of the aorta, which is the main artery that carries the blood from the heart to supply the needs of the body

aortic incompetence (aortic regurgitation, or leaky aortic valve) results from improper closing of the aortic valve that causes some of the blood to flow back to the left ventricle of the heart

arachnoiditis fibrosis (scarring) of the membrane covering the spinal cord and spinal nerve roots as they pass through the spinal canal. This results in entrapment of these nerve roots that may cause chronic back and leg pain and neurological dysfunction. It can occur following spinal surgery and has also been associated with the use of an X-ray contrast medium in the past. Very rarely, it can occur in the lower end of the spinal canal in AS without any apparent reason, and is the cause of **cauda equina syndrome** in this disease

arthralgia pain in one or more joints without any outward evidence of a joint abnormality

arthritis literally means inflammation of the joint and is used to refer to more than 100 joint diseases, some of which may also affect other regions of the body. The plural is **arthritidies**

arthritis mutilans an extremely destructive form of arthritis; the term is usually applied to a very severe form of psoriatic arthritis

arthrocentesis taking a sample of joint fluid out for testing, obtained by a needle puncture of the joint. Sometimes all of the joint fluid may be aspirated as a part of treatment

arthrodesis a surgically induced or spontaneous fusion of a joint

arthroplasty surgical procedure to alter a joint, e.g., its excision and replacement by an artificial joint

arthroscopy inspection of the inside of a joint, e.g., for performing joint surgery or obtaining a biopsy, usually through a fiber optic instrument called an **arthroscope**

artificial intelligence (AI) and **machine learning** methods can enable a computer, or a robot controlled by a computer, to perform tasks that normally require human intelligence and are therefore usually performed by humans

ASAS Health Index (ASAS HI) is an "all-in-one" index based on complaints of AS/axSpA patients about their pain, fatigue, and limitation in activities and social participation that are not adequately captured and assessed by using the currently used AS-specific questionnaires

autoimmune disease a disease in which the **immune system** attacks and destroys the body's own tissues that it mistakenly believes to be foreign

axial involvement or axial arthritis indicates involvement of the spine and/or neighbouring structures including the sacroiliac joints, the chest, and the "root" (appendicular) joints, i.e., the hip and shoulder joints

axial spondyloarthritis (axSpA) is an inflammatory arthritic disorder, primarily of the axial skeleton, that encompasses AS and non-radiographic axSpA (nr-axSpA)

Ayurveda the traditional Indian medical system, which claims that health is based on a harmonious relationship between three humors called "doshas," and disharmony results in disease

B cells (B lymphocytes) antibody-producing white blood cells, which mature in the bone marrow. The letter B originally came from bursa of Fabricius where B lymphocytes originate in chickens, but has subsequently been extended to imply the bone marrow

bamboo spine X-ray appearance of spine in advanced AS because of spinal fusion producing a bamboo-like appearance

BASDAI (Bath AS Disease Activity Index) was the first and a reliable, easy-to-use, and sensitive-to-change measure that was designed by medical professionals in conjunction with patients

BASFI (Bath AS Functional Index) is an easy, reliable, and sensitive-to-change method that assesses the degree of functional disability and coping skills

biologic agents (also known simply as **biologics** or **biologicals** or **biologic response modifiers** or **biologicals**) are drugs manufactured not by chemists but by living cells growing in big vats (containers) called bioreactor vats and tend to be quite expensive; they include TNF inhibitors, such as infliximab (Remicade®) and etanercept (Enbrel®)

biopsy removal of a small tissue specimen for examination

biosimilar is a biologic product "highly similar" to another already approved biologic, and has the same standards of pharmaceutical quality, safety, and efficacy. For the product to be labeled a "biosimilar" the manufacturer has to provide evidence that, among other things, their product is "highly similar" to an already-approved biological product. But the two products are not considered interchangeable and are therefore not called generics

Bisphosphonates drugs used to treat osteoporosis by inhibiting bone resorption

bone scan see DEXA

bowel a word commonly used for the small and large intestines (see **gut**; **large intestine**; **small intestine**)

brand name the brand name (trademark) of a drug is coined by the manufacturer in agreement with the regulating agencies, unlike the **generic name** which indicates its active ingredients. For example, celecoxib is the generic name for the drug whose brand name is Celebrex®. The brand name starts with a capital letter, but the generic name does not. Several brand-name drugs can have the same generic name if they contain the same active ingredient. Thus, Motrin® and Aleve® are both brand names for the generic drug ibuprofen

bursa a fluid-filled sac found between tissue planes over bony places that are subject to shearing forces, as over the elbows and knees. It is lined by synovium that secretes the lubricating fluid

bursitis an inflammation of a bursa

calcification deposition of chalky (calcific) material in tissue, leading to bone formation

Campylobacter a type of bacteria. Enteric infections with these bacteria can sometimes trigger reactive arthritis in susceptible individuals

cannabis is commonly known as **marijuana** and is closely related to hemp, a plant that has been used for its fiber since ancient times. Herbal cannabis is the dried cannabis plant or plant extracts in an oil or capsule form

capsule a thick membrane joining together ends of two adjacent bones to form a joint. Its inside is lined with synovium that forms the joint fluid

cartilage a tissue that covers the ends of bones to form a smooth shock-absorbing surface for joints, and results in very low-friction movement. Cartilage also occurs at other sites, such as the nose and the ears

cataract develops when the lens in the eye gradually becomes cloudy, with resultant impairment of light rays reaching the retina, and diminishes the eyesight

cauda equina syndrome some people with advanced AS on rare occasions may get this neurological condition resulting from gradual scarring at the lower end of the spine that entraps the lower spinal nerves. The name cauda equina means horsetail, so named because the lowermost spinal nerves slope downward as a bunch before they exit the vertebral column

CD4+ (CD8+) T lymphocytes these T cells carry a marker on the surface known as a cluster of differentiation (CD) marker which can be either CD4 or CD8. The CD4 + T cells, also known as **helper T cells,** help orchestrate the antibody responses, and the CD8 + T cells—also called **cytotoxic** (destructive cells) or **suppressor T cells**—are involved in cell-mediated immunity that targets infected cells

CDC Centers for Disease Control and Prevention in the United States

celiac disease inability to digest and absorb a protein found in wheat, resulting in poor absorption of nutrients from the foods because of damage to the lining of the small intestine; also called gluten intolerance or non-tropical sprue

central sensitization syndrome or simply **central sensitization** can be defined as a hypersensitivity to stimuli from things that are not typically painful. Also see **fibromyalgia**

cervical spine comprises 7 vertebrae in the neck

cervicitis inflammation of the cervix, the part of the uterus that protrudes into the vagina

chromosome a thread-like structure within the nucleus of a cell that contains the genes. There are 46 chromosomes in the nucleus of a human cell; 22 of them are in pairs that are given the numbers 1–22, and the remaining two are the X or Y chromosomes (sex chromosomes) that determine a person's sex—males have one X and one Y chromosomes, and females have two X chromosomes

Chlamydia trachomatis a bacterium that has a predilection to infect the genitourinary tract. Such an infection is the more commonly recognized initiator of reactive arthritis in the US

Clostridium difficile bacteria that are normally present in the large intestine, can cause a serious illness called pseudo-membranous colitis in people taking antibiotics, and can sometimes trigger reactive arthritis

coccyx is the lowest (final) segment of the spinal column, commonly called the 'tailbone'

collagen and **connective tissue** a set of fibrous proteins and supporting framework that form the main building blocks of the body, including the internal organs, ligaments, tendon, cartilage, bone, and skin

comorbidity is the simultaneous presence of more medical conditions or diseases in a patient

conjunctivitis commonly known as '**pink eye**'; it is an inflammation of the delicate outer membrane that lines the inside of the eyelids and the white of the eye

contracture arthritis or prolonged immobility can result in the involved joint becoming less freely moveable, associated with shortening and wasting of muscles

control group in clinical studies the control group, which is given either the standard treatment for a medical condition under study or an inactive substance (called a **placebo**), is compared with a group given an experimental treatment to find its efficacy for the disease under study

coping the psychological processes following any stressful situation

cortisone a natural hormone made by the adrenal gland. Sometimes wrongly used as a synonym for corticosteroids

corticosteroids a group of related compounds which, like cortisone, reduce inflammation and irritation caused by many disease processes, including many forms of arthritis, and skin and bowel diseases

costochondritis is the inflammation of the cartilage that connects ribs to the breastbone that results in local pain and tenderness

COVID-19 is the illness caused by infection with the original SARS-CoV2 stain of the virus and its subsequent new variants

C-reactive protein (CRP) its measurement in the blood can be used to detect or grade inflammation

Crohn's disease (CD) a chronic inflammatory bowel disease (also called ileitis or regional enteritis), that can affect the entire gastrointestinal tract, though it usually involves the lower small intestine (the ileum) and the adjacent part of the colon

cytokine a type of protein that is produced by certain immune and non-immune cells and acts as a messenger between cells, either stimulating or inhibiting the activity of various cells of the immune system. Examples include TNF and interferons. There is normally a very delicate balance among the various cytokines in the body

cytoplasm a liquid compartment in the cell, surrounding the central nucleus. The cytoplasm contains mitochondria and other structures or components responsible for normal protein formation, secretion, and other cell functions

dactylitis indicates diffuse inflammation of the fingers or toes taking on sausage-like appearance ("sausage digits")

DEXA or **DXA** stands for dual-energy X-ray absorption i.e., X-ray absorption at two different wavelengths (energies). It is a type of **bone scan** to measuring bone density for detection of osteoporosis at a much earlier stage as compared to a standard X-ray

disability in the context of health experience, a disability is a restriction or lack (resulting from an impairment) of ability to perform an activity in the manner or within the range considered normal

DISH or **diffuse idiopathic skeletal hyperostosis** is a type of degenerative arthritis that results in calcification and fusion of spinal ligaments (also see ankylosing hyperostosis)

disorder a synonym for disease

distal farther away from the trunk. For example, a hand is the distal end of an arm. The opposite is **proximal**

DMARDs (disease-modifying anti-rheumatic drugs), also abbreviated as conventional DMARDs (c-DMARDs), or conventional synthetic DMARDs (cs-DMARDs). The cs-DMARDs include drugs such as sulfasalazine and methotrexate. They are different from **biologic DMARDs** (**b-DMARDs**), such as the **TNF inhibitors** and **IL-17 inhibitors**. A new class of oral synthetic small molecular DMARDs, such as **tofacitinib** (**Xeljanz®**) and apremilast (Otezla®), are grouped under the term "**targeted synthetic DMARDs**" (**ts-DMARDs**) because they are developed to target a particular molecular structure

DNA (deoxyribonucleic acid) is a double-stranded, helical molecule that carries genetic information and consists of a string of four naturally occurring molecules (nucleotides) attached to sugar-phosphate backbone. The four nucleotides are assigned the letters A (adenine), T (thymine), G (guanine), and C (cytosine), and there are 6 billion letters in the human genome. DNA is primarily present within the nucleus of virtually all cell in plants and animals. It tells the cells exactly what to do and how to perform their functions and reproduce (also see **genome** and **epigenome**)

double-blinded a double-blinded trial produces more objective and unbiased results because neither the research investigators nor the study participants know who is receiving the investigational drug and who is receiving the placebo

duodenum the first part of the small intestine. An ulcer on its inner lining is called a **duodenal ulcer**

dowager's hump is the hump in the upper back (upper thoracic kyphosis) in an elderly person, mostly woman, with severe osteoporosis

dysentery an infectious disease of the intestine that causes bloody, mucus-filled diarrhea, which can be accompanied by abdominal pain or cramps, fever, and dehydration from excessive diarrhea. It is caused by enteric infections, usually with *Shigella*, and can sometimes trigger reactive arthritis in susceptible individuals

elimination diet requirement that certain foods should not be eaten

European Medicine Agency (EMA) in charge of protecting and promoting human and animal health by evaluating and supervising of medical products in Europe

enteritis an inflammation (irritation) of the small intestine

enthesis is the site of bony insertions of ligaments and tendons

enteropathic spondyloarthritis is a form of spondyloarthritis associated with **inflammatory bowel disease**

enthesitis is painful inflammation of an enthesis; the most typical enthesitis occurs in the heels at insertion sites of the Achilles tendon and plantar fascia

enthesopathy an all-inclusive term that covers all abnormalities of an enthesis (e.g., enthesitis is an inflammatory type of enthesopathy)

enzyme a protein that acts to promote or facilitate certain biochemical processes, e.g., many enzymes produced in the gut assist in digestion of food

epicondylitis enthesopathy at bony prominence (epicondyle) of the elbow; may occur on the medial (inner) side (golfer's elbow) or the lateral (outer) side (tennis elbow)

epigenome our DNA—our genome—tells the cells exactly what to do and how to perform their functions, and for that it requires the help from epigenome that includes chemical substances and also proteins (histones) that wrap around DNA to regulate how our genes function

erythrocyte sedimentation rate (ESR) a blood test commonly used to detect or grade inflammation

ESSG stands for **European SpA Study Group** that set up the ESSG criteria for SpA

esophagus the tube-like passage through which swallowed food travels from the mouth to the stomach

EULAR used to stand for **European League Against Rheumatism**, but in June 2021 the organization has now renamed itself as "**European Alliance of Associations for Rheumatology**"

extra-skeletal (or extra-musculoskeletal) manifestation of **AS/axSpA** include acute **anterior uveitis, psoriasis, and inflammatory bowel disease**

facet joints are located on either side of the back part of the spinal column that helps in rotation of the spine

familial a term used to indicate a disease or a trait (an inherited characteristic) which tends to affect more than one member in a family

fascia tough membrane that encloses muscles and other organs

fasciitis inflammation of the fascia

fibromyalgia a complex chronic painful condition, primarily occurring in women, characterized by widespread musculoskeletal pain and fatigue, and accompanied by tender points at defined locations, often associated with a non-restorative sleep pattern. Also see **pain sensitization syndrome**

fibrositis a term used interchangeably with **fibromyalgia**

folic acid and **folinic acid** are members of the vitamin B complex

food poisoning an acute food-borne gastrointestinal infection caused by food contaminated by harmful bacteria that results in symptoms such as diarrhea, abdominal discomfort or cramps, and fever

Forestier's disease see ankylosing hyperostosis and DISH

gastric ulcer an ulcer on the inner lining of the stomach

gastrointestinal tract is the alimentary tract, including esophagus, stomach, duodenum, ileum, large bowel, and rectum

gene (adj. genetic) is a segment of the DNA molecule responsible for making protein. It is the basic unit of heredity; all information in the genes (genetic information) is passed from parent to child. Genes influence how an organism looks and behaves

gene editing is the deliberate introduction of changes to genes by researchers

generic see generic name and **brand name**

genome is defined as the complete set of genetic material in a cell nucleus. We inherit one half of our genome from our mother and the other from our father. The study of this genetic inheritance housed within cells is known as **genomics**

genome-wide association studies (GWAS) have discovered 140 genetic variants, including HLA-B27, that together explain in excess of 30% of the total genetic risk for AS. HLA-B27 itself carries approximately 20% risk

generic name indicates a drugs active ingredient (also see **brand name** for further details)

genetic refers to any characteristic that is inherited

genetic counseling (or counselling) informing people about genetic facts that may guide them in making a decision based on knowledge of disease risk

Genetic marker a gene that is used to identify an individual disease or trait, or trace its inheritance within a family

genitourinary tract comprises the genitalia, the bladder, and the urethral tube through which the bladder empties

glaucoma means progressive loss of the field of vision, and it usually results from raised pressure in the eyeball

gut a word in common use to describe the large and small intestine (see **bowel, large intestine, small intestine**)

handicap in the context of health experience, a handicap is a disadvantage for a given individual, resulting from an impairment or a disability, that limits or prevents the fulfilment of a role that is normal (depending on age, sex, and social and cultural factors) for that individual

HAQ (Health Assessments Questionnaire) is a tool to evaluate functional disability that was later modified to a shorter version and also **HAQ-DI** (HAQ Disability Index

H2-blockers medicines such as cimetidine (Tagamet®), ranitidine (Zantac®), or famotidine (Pepcid®), used to treat acid indigestion, heartburn, and ulcer pain. They are so called because they act by blocking histamine-2 signals to reduce the amount of acid produced by the stomach

heartburn symptoms caused by stomach acid flowing back into the esophagus

Helicobacter pylori a corkscrew-shaped bacterium found in the stomach that can predispose to stomach and duodenal ulcers. Previously called *Campylobacter pylori*

heterozygote and **homozygote** an individual inherits a set of two **alleles** for each HLA locus from his or her parents. For instance, an individual may inherit HLA-B27 from one parent and HLA-B8 from the other. Most individuals do not inherit the same HLA from both parents and are said to be **heterozygotes**. Someone who inherits the same gene, e.g., HLA-B27, from both parents is **homozygous** for HLA-B27

HLA (human leucocyte antigens) These are cell surface proteins, detected by blood testing, that vary from person to person. They are also called tissue antigens or histocompatibility antigens because organ donors and recipients ideally must have compatible HLA; otherwise, the transplanted organ is recognized as non-self ("foreign") and is rejected. HLA are related to the workings of the immune system; they present self- and foreign-derived (e.g., viral) peptides (a few amino acids linked together) to T lymphocytes and other cells of the immune system that help the body fight illness. There are two broad types of HLA, called class I and class II, and their genes are located on chromosome 6; their locations or loci are given the letters A, B, C, D, and so on

HLA-B27 an HLA class I molecule that has been assigned the number 27; its gene is present at the B locus. There are quite a few HLA antigens that confer susceptibility to certain diseases, e.g., HLA-B27 increases risk of AS, and HLA-DR4 of rheumatoid arthritis

hydrotherapy physiotherapy in a pool (usually heated)

idiopathic of unknown cause or explanation

ileum a major part of the small intestine (see small intestine)

ilium (or **iliac bone**) major bony component of the pelvis. There is one on each side, joined to the sacrum via the right and left sacroiliac joints

immune can be used to mean an organism shows no impacts from a particular exposure, and generally it may be used that something cannot be hurt by a particular drug or disease

immunity indicates ability to ward off a particular infection, and it can be innate (one is born with it) or acquired during life experience

impairment in the context of health experience, an impairment is any loss or abnormality of psychological, physiological, or anatomical structure or function

incidence the rate of occurrence of some event, such as the number of individuals who get a disease divided by a total given population, per unit of time (usually per year), i.e., how often a new case is diagnosed. It is usually stated as the number of cases observed per 100,000 individuals

inflammation a typical reaction of tissues to injury or disease, usually marked by four signs: pain, swelling, redness, and heat. It may be acute (as in a burn or in gouty arthritis) or chronic (as in AS, rheumatoid arthritis or chronic infections such as tuberculosis)

inflammatory bowel disease (IBD) a chronic (long-lasting) inflammatory disease of the gut, fairly evenly split between ulcerative colitis (UC) and Crohn's disease (CD)

interferons are a group of signalling proteins released by a virus-infected cell causing nearby cells to enhance their anti-viral defences.

interleukin-17 (abbreviated as IL-17) is a pro-inflammatory cytokine that plays a critical role, along with TNF, in patients suffering from SpA, especially AS and PsA

IL-23 is another pro-inflammatory cytokine

IL-17 inhibitors secukinumab (Cosentyx®) and ixekizumab (Taltz®) are approved by the FDA and the European Medicines Agency (EMA) for the treatment of adult patients with active AS/axSpA, psoriasis and PsA, but they are not effective for treatment of IBD

IL-23 inhibitors are approved for the treatment of moderate to severe plaque psoriasis and PsA. They have unprecedented efficacy of even complete skin clearance of psoriasis in a high percentage of patients, compared to TNF inhibitors

intermittent fasting is a dietary intervention that focuses on the timing when a person can eat within a day or within a week. The two prominent patterns are 'alternate day fasting' and 'time-restricted eating'

internist a doctor specializing in internal medicine (not requiring surgery)

intervertebral disc acts as a shock absorber located between two adjacent vertebral bodies

intestine also called bowel or gut (see **large intestine, small intestine**)

intestinal flora bacteria and other organisms that normally reside in the intestine

intestinal mucosa surface lining of the intestines where the absorption of nutrients takes place

intra-articular into or within a joint, e.g., intra-articular injection

irritable bowel syndrome is an intestinal disorder that is not well understood and is associated with belly pain, bloating, excessive gas (flatus) and episodes of constipation and diarrhea

iritis is an older term replaced by '**uveitis**'

JAK inhibitors (JAKi) are a class of drugs that are taken as tablets, and two of them (**tofacitinib** and **upadacitinib**) have been approved for the treatment of AS and PsA

joint is the place where two bones meet. Most joints are composed of cartilage, joint space, fibrous capsule, joint lining (synovium), and ligaments

juvenile chronic arthritis occurring in children 16 years of age or less, that has been present for at least 3 months, and for which no other cause is obvious. It is now preferably called **juvenile idiopathic arthritis**

keratoderma blennorrhagica rash on palms of the hands and soles of the feet which may occur in reactive arthritis (Reiter's syndrome); it can resemble a form of psoriasis

kyphosis forward stooping (bowing) of the spine ('humpback' deformity)

large intestine part of the intestine that changes stool from a liquid to a solid form by absorbing water. It is 1.5 meters (5 feet) long and is often simply called the colon, but in fact includes the appendix, cecum, colon, and rectum

leukocyte white blood cell, part of the immune system

ligament stretchy tough band of cord-like tissue that connects bones together, and confers stability by restraining excessive joint movement

limb girdle joints hip and shoulder joints

locus precise location of a gene on a chromosome

long COVID is a term commonly used to describe symptoms that continue or develop after acute COVID-19. The WHO has renamed it "post COVID-19 condition" and have estimated that 10–20% of COVID-19 patients experience such lingering symptoms

lymphocyte a type of white blood cell present in the blood, lymph, and lymphoid tissues; primarily responsible for immune responses (see also **B lymphocytes; CD4+ (CD8+) T lymphocytes; T lymphocytes**)

macrophage a relatively large immune system cell that devours invading bacteria and other intruders and stimulates other immune cells by presenting them with small pieces of the invaders. They can sometimes harbor some of the infecting microbes like HIV without being killed, and thus act as a reservoir of such viruses

magnetic resonance imaging (MRI) a method of taking better and clearer pictures of the soft tissues in the body than those obtained by X-rays, and without radiation

marijuana is also known as cannabis. Medical marijuana specifically refers to its use for medicinal purposes, and it contains specific amounts of molecules called tetrahydrocannabinol (**THC**) and cannabidiol (**CBD**)

medial on the inside (as opposed to **lateral**); not to be confused with the **median** nerve which is compressed in carpal tunnel syndrome

medical alert and personalized information cards contain concise health-related information about the patient

methotrexate (MTX) a drug which is used in low doses for the treatment of inflammatory disorders, including various types of inflammatory arthritis. (See also **slow-acting anti-rheumatic drugs**)

microbiome refers to the trillions of living microorganisms (microbes), such as bacteria, viruses and fungi, that live in a balanced way on our skin (skin microbiome) and in our gut (gut microbiome). Only a fraction of them have been fully identified and cultured in research labs. Microbial cells far outnumber human cells and that implies that we are more microbe than human

monoclonal antibodies artificially produced antibodies used in research and also for treatment of some diseases. They are produced in a cell culture (clone) by multiplying one single mother cell thus having the same properties (very pure antibody)

MRI See magnetic resonance imaging

nucleus the central controlling structure within a living cell that contains the genetic codes (in chromosomes) for maintaining life systems of the cell and for issuing commands for cell growth and reproduction

nausea the feeling of wanting to throw up (vomit)

neurohormones biochemical substances made by tissue in the body's nervous system that can change the function or structure, or direct the activity of tissues or organs, e.g., neurotransmitters

neurological relating to the body's nervous system, which oversees and controls all body functions

neurotransmitters biochemical substances that stimulate or inhibit nerve impulses in the brain that relay information about external stimuli and sensations, such as pain

National Institute of Health (NIH) is the world's foremost medical research center, and its many websites provide the latest and most useful research and health related information

National Institute for Health and Clinical Excellence (NICE) publishes guidelines for the use of health technologies, clinical practice, health promotion and social care services of the UK's NHS

National Health Service (NHS) is the UK's biggest health service and its website provides very useful information from the government-funded health service

neutrophils are part of the innate immune defense system and from 40% to 70% of white blood cells (WBC) in our body

NK (natural killer) cells non-specific lymphocytes like killer T cells that attack and kill cancer and infected cells. They are natural killers because they do not need to recognize a specific antigen to attack and kill

NSAIDs (non-steroidal anti-inflammatory drugs) non-cortisone, non-addictive (non-narcotic) drugs that reduce pain and inflammation and are therefore used in the treatment of pain and arthritis

occiput to wall distance measures the degree of fixed forward stooping of the neck

oligoarthritis is defined as inflammation of up to four joints; if more joints are involved, then the term **polyarthritis** is used

onycholysis nail abnormality and discoloration seen in psoriasis and reactive arthritis; may be accompanied by pitting of the nail in psoriasis

Osgood–Schlatter's disease a childhood condition of the site of attachment of the patellar (kneecap) tendon into the tibial tubercle, a bony prominence an inch or so below the kneecap. It results in localized pain and tenderness that can sometimes be confused with enthesitis at this site seen in some children with juvenile AS and related diseases

osteitis condensans ilii increased bone density (sclerosis) at the sacral side of the sacroiliac joint that is of unknown cause and is usually without symptoms. Its X-ray appearance can be confused with sacroiliitis

osteoarthritis (osteoarthrosis) degenerative disorder of joints, most often from disease in the spine and in the weight-bearing joints (knees and hips). Normally seen with aging, but can occur prematurely due to various reasons, for instance after an injury to a joint. Also known as **degenerative joint disease,** it can cause joint pain, loss of function, reduced joint motion, and deformity

osteomalacia bone-thinning disorder resulting from deficiency of vitamin D. This term can be mistaken for osteoporosis. The childhood form of osteomalacia is called **rickets**

osteophyte bony outgrowth (seen on X-ray) at joint margin of an osteoarthritic joint, or in degenerative disc disease

osteoporosis a disease characterized by reduction in mineral content usually seen with aging, but also in connection with certain conditions such as paralysis, or due to prolonged use of certain drugs, such as corticosteroids

Paget's disease is also called **osteitis deformans** and is characterized by accelerated bone turnover, resulting in the involved bone becoming enlarged but weak and fragile. The bone also feels warmer to touch due to increased blood supply

pain is an unpleasant sensory and emotional experience associated with, or resembling that associated with, actual or potential tissue damage

pathogenesis process of development of a disease

patient reported outcome (PRO) measures (PROM) are defined as any reports that report the status of patient's health condition that comes directly from the patient. Examples include BASDAI, BASFI, HAQ, and many others

pauciarthritis same as oligoarthritis

pelvis the bony structures in the lowest part of the trunk. The term **pelvic** is used for anything that belongs or refers to the pelvis

peptic ulcer a sore in the lining of the stomach (**gastric ulcer**) or duodenum (**duodenal ulcer**). The word peptic refers to the stomach and the duodenum, where pepsin is present, an enzyme that breaks down proteins. An ulcer can sometimes occur in the lower part of the esophagus in association with heartburn

peptide a few amino acids linked together. Proteins are made of multiple peptides linked together

peripheral joint involvement implies arthritis of limb joints. The hip and shoulder joints ("root joints") are excluded because they form part of the axial skeleton

placebo originally a Latin word meaning "I will please." Now used for inactive substance (sham) given to participants of a research study to test the efficacy of another substance or treatment. In short-term clinical trials, many of the most valued drugs in clinical use are only about 25% more effective than placebo. Scientists often have to compare the effects of active and inactive substances to learn more about how the active substance affects participants; in such studies called randomized placebo controlled trials (RCT) both doctor and patient are unaware of who is receiving the active or inactive substance. Such studies are known as **double blind placebo-controlled** studies

polyarthralgia pains in many joints (conventionally refers to more than four joints) without signs of inflammation in the symptomatic joints

polyarthritis inflammation in many joints; conventionally in more than four joints

prebiotics are sources of indigestible fibers (or roughage) that provide no calories and prevent constipation, but some of the gut bacteria (gut microbiome) can feed on them and increase bacterial variety

probiotics are live yeast and certain human derived bacteria that contribute to digestive health. Yogurt and kefir are widely regarded as the best probiotics. Other non-diary probiotics include sauerkraut, kimchi, and Japanese natto

preclinical diagnosis of a genetic disease before there are any symptoms or signs

prevalence the observed number of people in population affected with a particular disease or condition at a given time, usually stated as a percentage. It can be thought of as a snapshot of all existing cases at a specified time

prognosis the probable end-result or outcome of a disease

protein a large molecule composed of amino acids. Proteins form the essential components of the body tissue

proton pump inhibitors a group of drugs used to treat heartburn and peptic ulcer disease. These include omeprazole (Prilosec®), esomeprazole (Nexium®), and pansoprazole (Prevacid®)

prospective, randomized, double blind study clinical trial or study in which the method of data analysis is specified in a protocol before the study is begun (prospective). Patients are randomly assigned to receive either the study drug or an alternative treatment, and neither the patient nor the doctor conducting the study knows which treatment is being given to which patient (see also **placebo**)

proximal the part of a limb that is closest to the trunk. For example, the shoulder joint forms the proximal end of the upper extremity (opposite of **distal**)

psoriasis a common chronic skin disease, more common in whites (2% of the population) than in other racial groups, in which red flaky lesions occur—often on the elbows and knees, or in the scalp. May cause nail abnormalities and may lead to arthritis

psoriatic arthritis (PsA) is a form of spondyloarthritis that is associated with psoriasis

pulmonary a medical term for the lungs

Qi Chinese term for vital energy or life force. Pronounced "chee" (see **acupuncture**)

radiography/radiograph/radiogram/radiological or roentgenography the method of taking a picture with the help of X-rays, and the terms radiograph or simply X-ray are used for the resulting picture. Radiogram is the correct name for an image taken by radiography

radon use of combined low-dose radon/hyperthermia "baths" in mines are still used in some German-speaking countries but are not advised

randomized, double-blind, placebo-controlled, multicenter trial is a clinical trial in which patients have been randomly assigned to receive either the study drug or the alternative treatment under study. Neither the patient nor the doctor conducting the study knows which treatment is being given; the alternative to the study drug is a placebo; and the study is conducted at several research centers

range of motion the extent to which a joint can go through all of its normal movements. Range-of-motion exercises help increase or maintain flexibility and movement in muscles, tendons, ligaments, and joints

reactive arthritis results from infectious trigger elsewhere in the body, i.e., there is no infection in the inflamed joint. The commonest type is HLA B27-related and may follow certain types of infections in the gut or the genito-urinary tract. Another example is rheumatic fever triggered by strep infection in the throat

RAPID3 (Routine Assessment of Patient Index Data 3) is a pooled index of 3 patient-reported measures: pain, physical abilities (function), and patient global estimate of status

Reiter's syndrome a form of HLA B27-related reactive arthritis with a classical triad of arthritis, conjunctivitis, and urethritis, with or without other features of spondyloarthritis. The term **reactive arthritis** is now used more commonly to describe this condition

rheumatic fever a form of reactive arthritis triggered by streptococcal sore throat. Its features include very painful joint inflammation (arthritis). It is now uncommon in developed countries but still occurs commonly in other parts of the world. It can cause inflammation and scarring of heart valves (rheumatic heart disease)

rheumatoid arthritis a chronic systemic disease that causes inflammatory changes in the synovium, or joint lining, that result in pain, stiffness, swelling, and ultimately loss of function and deformities of the affected joints due to destruction of the cartilage and adjacent bone. The disease can also affect other parts of the body. In the past it was also called **chronic polyarthritis**. It is more common in women than men, and at least 70% of patients show a positive blood test for **rheumatoid factor**

rheumatologist a doctor (board-certified internist or pediatrician) who has had specialized training in diagnosing and treating disorders that affect the joints, muscles, tendons, ligaments, connective tissue, and bones

roentgenography see **radiography**

sacroiliac joint a joint, one on either side, in the lower back, between the sacrum in the middle and the ilium (a major part of the pelvic bone) on both sides (see Figure 1.4)

sacroiliitis inflammation of the sacroiliac joint; bilateral sacroiliitis is a hallmark of AS

sacrum major bony component of the pelvis, shaped like a wedge on which the spine rests. It forms a joint with ilium, one on each side, via the right and left sacroiliac joints

Salmonella a group of bacteria comprising many different types that may cause intestinal infection and diarrhea called **salmonellosis**, which includes typhoid fever. Enteric infections with *Salmonella, Shigella, Yersinia*, or *Campylobacter* are the most common triggers for reactive arthritis, especially in some developing parts of the world

SAPHO syndrome so named because of its salient features: synovitis, acne, palmoplantar pustulosis, hyperostosis, aseptic osteomyelitis. It causes aseptic (no evidence of infection) bone necrosis at multiple sites that can include the sacroiliac joints or the spine. It is known by many different names, but SAPHO syndrome is the most common

sausage digit finger or toe that is diffusely swollen because of tenosynovitis; usually seen in psoriatic and reactive arthritis. It is also called dactylitis

Scheuermann's disease a non-inflammatory spinal disease that occurs in adolescence and affects the thoracic spine, especially the discs. Often painless, but can result in a stooped back

Schöber's test or Schoeber test is used to detect the ability to bend forward (flexibility) of the lumbar spine (see Figure 8.1g)

scoliosis a non-inflammatory rotational deformity of the spine; results in a lateral curvature

selective estrogen receptor modulators (SERM) a class of drugs used in the treatment of osteoporosis; they mimic the effect of estrogen but in a tissue-selective manner

septic arthritis bacterial infection of one or more joints; requires urgent diagnosis and treatment

seronegative arthritis an arthritis that is not associated with the presence of an autoantibody called **rheumatoid factor** in the blood. Only about 25% of people with rheumatoid arthritis (RA) are seronegative. On the other hand, most people with AS and related SpA lack this autoantibody, and therefore these diseases are examples of seronegative arthritis

Shigella a group of bacteria that can cause an illness called **shigellosis**, with high fever and acute diarrhea, sometimes mixed with blood (dysentery). Enteric infections with *Shigella* can trigger reactive arthritis

shingles (herpes zoster) a viral infection (varicella zoster virus) that causes painful rash on one side of the face or the body. A chickenpox vaccine in childhood or a shingles vaccine (named Shingrix®) as an adult can minimize the risk of developing shingles

sibling brother or sister

skeletal muscles are those that move the bony skeleton, i.e., provide movement at the joints

slit lamp an instrument used by eye specialists (opthalmologists) to look for inflammation or other diseases inside the eye

slow-acting anti-rheumatic drugs (SAARDs), also called symptom-modifying drugs (**SMARDs**), such as sulfasalazine and methotrexate. Any benefit from these drugs takes some time to manifest itself, hence the name. Unlike **NSAIDs**, these drugs are not pain relievers, but they will help relieve pain if they can first heal or control the underlying inflammation. Also see **DMARDs**

small intestine (or small bowel) is the tubular organ, almost 7 meters (22 feet) long, where most of the food is digested. It is made up of three parts: the **duodenum** (which is attached to the stomach), **jejunum,** and **ileum** (which ends in the large intestine)

spinal column or vertebral column comprises the vertebral bodies and surrounding ligaments and muscles that keep us upright and enclose the spinal cord

spondylitis literally means inflammation of the spine, and is best exemplified by ankylosing spondylitis (AS)

spondyloarthritis (previously called **spondyloarthopathy** or **spondyloarthropathies**) encompasses AS and related diseases that share many clinical features, and occur much more often in people who carry the HLA-B27 gene

spondylolisthesis a loss of spinal column alignment that results from one vertebra slipping forward on top of another

spondylosis non-inflammatory degenerative (wear and tear) disease of the spinal column as we get older, such as degenerative disc disease

steroids see **corticosteroids**

stomach ulcer an open sore in the lining of the stomach. Also called **gastric ulcer**

sulfasalazine see **slow-acting anti-rheumatic drugs**

syndesmophytes are ligamentous bone deposits (ossification) producing fine bony bridging between adjacent vertebral bodies at the margin of the vertebrae, characteristic of AS. They are vertically orientated, unlike osteophytes (seen in degenerative disc disease), which grow horizontally

syndrome a complex of signs and symptoms that when occurring together suggest a particular disease

synovium a thin membrane (normally one or two cell layers thick) lining the inside of the joint capsule. It produces **synovial fluid** for lubrication and nourishment of the joint cartilage

synovitis inflammation of the joints resulting from inflamed synovium; this results in joint inflammation (arthritis)

systemic implies involvement of a whole system, e.g., systemic versus localized inflammation

T cell (or **T lymphocyte**) T stands for the thymus, where T lymphocytes mature. T cells are white blood cells that play a critical role in immune response, but, unlike B lymphocytes, do not produce antibodies (immunoglobulins). There are two main subtypes: the **CD4 + helper T cells** and the **CD8 + cytotoxic or suppressor T cells**

Tai Chi a traditional Chinese mind–body relaxation exercise consisting of 108 intricate exercise sequences performed in a slow relaxed manner over a 30-minute period

temporo-mandibular joint (TMJ) the jaw joint

tendon a tough cord or band of fibrous tissue by which muscles are attached to bone

tendinitis (tendonitis) inflammation of a tendon

tenosynovitis an inflammation extending to the sheaths containing lubricating fluid that surrounds the tendon

TENS (transcutaneous electrical nerve stimulation) a type of therapy used to relieve pain that involves passing electricity to nerve cells through electrodes placed on the skin

THA (Total Hip Arthroplasty or **THR (Total Hip Replacement))** means surgical total hip joint replacement

thromboembolism obstruction of a blood vessel by a blood clot (or a piece of it) that gets dislodged from another site in the circulation. For example, dislodging of a blood clot from a vein in the leg and resulting in obstruction of blood vessels in the lung is called pulmonary (lung) thromboembolism

TKA (Total Knee Arthroplasty) means surgical total knee joint replacement

TMJ temporo-mandibular joint or jaw joint

TNF (tumor necrosis factor) a cytokine (messenger protein) that plays a key role in the body's immune response by promoting inflammation, controlling the production of other pro-inflammatory molecules, and helping the cells heal or repair themselves. It attaches to a cell surface protein called "TNF receptor" to exert its effect on the cell

TNF inhibitors (TNFi) or TNF blockers are very effective for decreasing symptoms and signs of AS/axSpA, some of the other forms of SpA, RA, psoriasis, and inflammatory bowel disease. They include infliximab (Remicade®), etanercept (Enbrel®), adalimumab (Humira®), certolizumab (Cimzia®), and golimumab (Simponi®)

tofacitinib (Xeljanz®) is one of the JAK-inhibitors that is approved for the treatment of adults with active PsA and AS who have had an inadequate response or intolerance to one or more TNF-inhibitors

trademark or registered trademark is ®, and see brand name for further details

tumor necrosis factor—see TNF

tumor suppressor gene p53 is called "guardian of the genome" because it prevents genome mutation (alteration)

traditional Chinese medicine (TCM) is an ancient Chinese system of medicine that includes meditation, herbal and nutritional therapy, restorative physical exercises and massage, and acupuncture. (See also **acupuncture, alternative healthcare,** and **complementary remedies**)

twin's concordance rate is the ratio number of twin-pairs affected with a disease or condition over the total number of such pairs studied

ulcer is a sore on the skin surface or on the inside lining of a body part, such as the mouth, stomach, or the gut (intestinal tract)

ulcerative colitis (UC) is an inflammatory disease of the inner lining of the gut that usually involves the colon or rectum. (See also **inflammatory bowel disease (IBD)**)

upadacitinib (Rinvoq®) belongs to a class of drugs called JAK inhibitors approved for the treatment of adults with active nr-axSpA, AS, and PsA

urethritis an inflammatory condition of the urethra (the tube through which the urine travels from the bladder to the outside during urination)

ustekinumab (Stelara®) is an IL-12/IL-23 inhibitor that is FDA approved for the treatment of psoriasis, psoriatic arthritis (PsA), ulcerative colitis (UC), and Crohn's disease (CD)

uveitis—see acute anterior uveitis

vaccine is a biologic preparation that provides and/or enhances immunity to a particular infectious agent. **Vaccination** is the process of administering a vaccine

vertebrae are the bones that form the vertebral (spinal) column

WBC (white blood cells) see neutrophils

Yersinia a group of bacteria comprising many different types that may cause intestinal infection and diarrhea. Enteric infections with *Yersinia*, *Salmonella*, *Shigella*, or *Campylobacter* are the most common triggers for reactive arthritis

Appendix 3

Further reading

Recent books (since 2002) on AS/axSpA by the author

Khan MA, Akkoc N. ANKYLOSING SPONDYLITIS-AXIAL SPONDYLOARTHRITIS. 2nd Edition, Professional Communications Inc. (PCI). West Islip, NY. 2021, 436 pages. ISBN: 978-1-943236-30-5.

Mease P, Khan MA (Eds). AXIAL SPONDYLOARTHRITIS. Elsevier. 2020, 294 pages. ISBN: 978-0-323:56800-5.

Khan MA: ANKYLOSING SPONDYLITIS-AXIAL SPONDYLOARTHRITIS. 1st Edition. Professional Communications Inc. (PCI). West Islip, NY. 2016. 333 pages. ISBN: 978-1-943236-08-4.

Khan MA: ANKYLOSING SPONDYLITIS. Oxford University Press, New York, NY. 2009, 147 pages. ISBN: 978-0-19-536807-9.

Khan MA: 1st Edition. ANKYLOSING SPONDYLITIS: THE FACTS. Oxford University Press, Oxford, UK, 2002; 193 pages. ISBN: 0-19-263282-5

Portuguese translation was published in 2004

Japanese translation was published in 2008

Persian (Farsi) *translation* was published in 2008

Spanish translation was published in 2012

Khan MA: Guest Editor. Ankylosing Spondylitis: Burden of Illness; Diagnosis, and Effective Treatment. *J Rheumatol* Suppl 2006; Sep; 78:1–33

References for further reading

1. Akkoc N and Khan MA. "JAK inhibitors for axial spondyloarthritis: What the future holds?" *Curr Rheumatol Rep.* 2021 28 Apr;23(6):34. doi:10.1007/s11926-021-01001-1.

2. Akkoc N and Khan MA. "Epidemiology of axial spondyloarthritis" in Mease P and Khan MA (eds), *Axial Spondyloarthritis.* Elsevier, 2019, 31–56.

3. Akkoc N and Khan MA. "Is axial spondyloarthritis more common than rheumatoid arthritis?" *Curr Rheumatol Rep.* 2020;22:54. https://doi.org/10.1007/s11926-020-00934-3.

4. Akkoc N, van der Linden S, and Khan MA. "Ankylosing spondylitis and symptom-modifying versus disease-modifying therapy" *Best Pract Res Clin Rheumatol.* 2006 June;20(3):539–57.

5. Akkoc N and Khan MA. "ASAS classification criteria for axial spondyloarthritis: Time to modify" *Clin Rheumatol.* 2016;35(6):1415–23.

6. Akkoc N, Yarkan H, Kenar G, and Khan MA. "Ankylosing spondylitis: HLA-B*27 Positive versus HLA-B*27 negative disease" *Curr Rheumatol Rep.* 2017 May;19(5):26. doi:10.1007/s11926-017-0654-8.

7. Antonelli M, Khan MA, and Magrey MN. "Differential events between TNF-a inhibitors and IL-17 axis inhibitors for the treatment of spondyloarthritis" *Curr Treat Options Rheumatol.* 2015;1(2):239–54.

8. Baumberger H and Khan MA. "Gradual progressive change to equal prevalence of ankylosing spondylitis among males and females in Switzerland: Data from the Swiss Ankylosing Spondylitis Society (SVMB)" *Ann Rheum Dis.* 2017;76(Suppl 2):929.

9. Baumberger H, Giovanni ME, and Khan MA. "Description of 'panoramic field' for assessment of impaired ability of ankylosing spondylitis patients to fully see their surroundings despite having normal field of vision" *Rheuma Schweiz Fachzeitschrift.* 2019;6:30–4.

10. Bidad K, Gracey E, Hemington K, *et al.* "Pain in ankylosing spondylitis: a neuroimmune collaboration" *Nat Rev Rheumatol.* 2017;13:410–20. <https://doi.org/10.1038/nrrheum.2017.92>.

11. Bittar M, Yong, Magrey M, and Khan MA. "Worldwide differences in clinical phenotypes of axial spondyloarthritis" *Curr Rheumatol Rep.* 2021;23:76. doi.org/10.1007/s11926-021-01043-5.

12. Cherqaoui B. "Axial spondyloarthritis: Emerging drug targets" *Expert Opin Ther Targets.* 2021 Aug;25(8):633–44. doi:10.1080/14728222.2021.1973429. doi:10.1080/14728222.2021.1973429.

13. Chetrit M, Kapadia S, and Khan MA. State of the art management of aortic valve disease in ankylosing spondylitis. *Curr Rheumatol Rep.* 2020 May 14;22(6):23. doi:10.1007/s11926-020-00898-4

14. Costantino F, Talpin A, Said-Nahal R, *et al.* "Prevalence of spondyloarthritis in reference to HLA-B27 in the French population: results of the GAZEL cohort" *Ann Rheum Dis.* 2015;74:689–93. doi:10.1136/annrheumdis-2013-204436.

15. Dickhoff T, Hermann KG, and Lambert RG. "Future of low-dose computed tomography and dual-energy computed tomography in axial spondyloarthritis" *Curr Rheumatol Rep.* 2022 (in press)

16. Dong TA, Sandesara PB, Dhindsa DS, *et al.* "Intermittent fasting: a heart healthy dietary pattern?" *Am J Med.* 2020 Aug;133(8):901–7. doi:10.1016/j.amjmed.2020.03.030.

17. D'Silva KM and Wallace ZS. "COVID-19 and disease-modifying anti-rheumatic drugs" *Curr Rheumatol Rep.* 2021;23:28. https://doi.org/10.1007/s11926-021-00998-9.

18. Editorial. "Understanding long COVID: A modern medical challenge" *Lancet.* 2021 28 Aug;398(10302):725. doi:10.1016/S0140-6736(21)01900-0.

19. Elyan M and Khan MA. "The role of non-steroidal anti-inflammatory medications and exercise in the treatment of ankylosing spondylitis" *Curr Rheumatol Rep.* 2006;8:255–9.

20. Feldtkeller E, Bruckel J, and Khan MA. "Scientific contributions of ankylosing spondylitis patient advocacy groups" *Curr Opin Rheumatol.* 2000 Jul;12(4):239–47. doi:10.1097/00002281-200007000-00002. PMID: 10910174.

21. Feldtkeller E, Khan MA, van der Heijde D, van der Linden S, and Braun J. "Age at disease onset and diagnosis delay in HLA-B27 negative vs. positive patients with ankylosing spondylitis" *Rheumatol Intl.* 2003 Mar;23(2):61–6. doi:10.1007/s00296-002-0237-4. Epub 2002 Sep 3. PMID: 12634937.

22. Goldberg DS and McGee SJ. "Pain as a global public health priority." *BMC Public Health*. 2011 Oct 6;11:770. doi:10.1186/1471-2458-11-770. PMID: 21978149; PMCID: PMC3201926.

23. Gracey E, Vereecke L, McGovern D, *et al.* "Revisiting the gut–joint axis: Links between gut inflammation and spondyloarthritis." *Nat Rev Rheumatol*. 2020 Aug;16(8):415–33. doi:10.1038/s41584-020-0454-9. Epub 2020 Jul 13. PMID: 32661321.

24. Gregory WJ, Kaur J, Bamford S, *et al.* "A survey of diagnostic delay in axial spondyloarthritis across two National Health Service (NHS) rheumatology services." *Cureus*. 30 Mar 2022;14(3):e23670. doi:10.7759/cureus.23670.

25. Han Q, Zheng Z, Zhang K, *et al.* "A comprehensive assessment of hip damage in ankylosing spondylitis, especially early features." *Front Immunol*. 2021 Mar 24. <https//doi.org/10.3389/fimmu.2021.668969>.

26. Huwang MC, Lee MJ, Gensler LS, *et al.* "Identifying trajectories of radiographic spinal disease in ankylosing spondylitis: A 15-year follow up study of the PSOAS cohort." *Rheumatology*. 2021. <https://doi.org/10.1093/rheumatology/keab661>.

27. Ji X, Hu L, Wang Y, *et al.* "'Mobile health' for the management of spondyloarthritis, and its application in China." *Curr Rheumatol Rep*. 2019 Nov 19;21(11):61. <https://doi.org/10.1007/s11926-019-0860-7>.

28. Jovani V, Blasco-Blasco M, Ruiz-Cantero MT, and Pascual E. "Understanding how the diagnostic delay of spondyloarthritis differs between women and men: A systematic review and meta-analysis." *J Rheumatol*. 2017;44(2):174–83. doi:10.3899/jrheum.160825.

29. Kahn M-F and Khan MA. "SAPHO syndrome." *Ballière's Clinical Rheumatology* 1994;8:333–62.

30. Khan MA. "A worldwide overview—The epidemiology of HLA-B27 and associated spondyloarthritides" in Calin A and Taurog J (eds), *The Spondyloarthritidies*. Oxford: Oxford University Press, 1998, 17–26.

31. Khan MA. "HLA-B27and its subtypes in world populations." *Curr Opin Rheumatol*. 1995;7:263–9.

32. Khan MA. "My self-portrait." *Clin Rheumatol*. 2001;20:1–2.

33. Khan MA and Khan MK. "Survival among patients with ankylosing spondylitis: a life-table analysis." *J Rheumatol*. 1981;8:86–90.

34. Khan MA. "Back and neck pain" in Bone RC (ed), *Current Practice of Medicine*. Edinburgh: Churchill Livingstone, 1996, 1–14.

35. Khan MA. "Spondyloarthropathies" in Hunder G (ed), *Atlas of Rheumatology*. Philadelphia, PA: Current Science, 2005, 151–80.

36. Khan MA, Garcia-Kutzbach A, and Espinoza LR. "Treatment of ankylosing spondylitis: A critical reappraisal of nonsteroidal anti-inflammatory drugs and corticosteroids." *Am J Med Sciences*. 2012 May;343(5):350–2.

37. Khan MA, Haroon M, and Rosenbaum JT. "Acute anterior uveitis and spondyloarthritis: More than meets the eye." *Curr Rheumatol Rep*. 2015;17(9):536. doi:10.1007/s11926-015-0536-x.

38. Khan MA. "Accomplishments of Heinz Baumberger PhD: a remarkable patient with ankylosing spondylitis for 72 years." *Clin Rheumatol*. 2016;35(6):1637–41.

39. Khan MA. "An update on the genetic polymorphism of *HLA-B*27* with 213 alleles encompassing 160 subtypes (and Still Counting)." *Curr Rheumatol Rep*. 2017 Feb;19(2):9. doi:10.1007/s11926-017-0640-1.

40. Khan MA and van der Linden S. "Axial spondyloarthritis: A better name for an old disease: A step toward uniform reporting" *ACR Open Rheumatology*. 2019. doi:10.1002/acr2.11044.

41. Khan MA and van der Linden SM. "A wider spectrum of spondyloarthropathies" *Semin Arthritis Rheum*. 1990;20:107–13.

42. Khan MA. "Update on spondyloarthropathies" *Ann Intern Med*. 2002;136:896–907.

43. Khan MA. "Thoughts concerning the early diagnosis of ankylosing spondylitis and related diseases" *Clin Exp Rheumatol*. 2002;20(Suppl 28):S6–S10.

44. Khan MA, van der Linden SM, Kushner I, *et al*. "Spondylitic disease without radiological evidence of sacroiliitis in relatives of HLA-B27 positive patients" *Arthritis Rheum*. 1985;28:40–3.

45. Khan MA and Khan MK. "Diagnostic value of HLA-B27 testing in ankylosing spondylitis and Reiter's syndrome" *Ann Intern Med*. 1982;96:70–6.

46. Khan MA. "Patient-doctor" *Ann Intern Med*. 2000;133:233–5.

47. Khan MA. "Patient's perspective" in van Royen BJ and Dijkmans BAC (eds), *Ankylosing Spondylitis Diagnosis and Management*. New York, NY: Taylor and Francis, 2006, 95–7.

48. Khan MA. "Clinical features of axial spondylorthritis" in Inman R and Sieper J (eds), *Oxford Textbook of Axial Spondyloarthritis*. Oxford: Oxford University Press, 2016, 91–100.

49. Kieskamp SC, Pap D, Carbo MJG, *et al*. "Central sensitization has major impact on quality of life in patients with axial spondyloarthritis" *Semin Arthritis Rheum*. 2021. <https://doi.org/10.1016/j.semarthrit.2021.11.006>.

50. Kiltz U, van der Heijde D, Boonen A, *et al*. "Development of a health index in patients with ankylosing spondylitis (ASAS HI): Final result of a global initiative based on the ICF guided by ASAS" *Ann Rheum Dis*. 2015;74(5):830–5.

51. Kiltz U, Wendling D, and Braun J. "ASAS Health Index: the 'all in one' for spondyloarthritis evaluation" *J Rheumatol*. 2020;47(10):1457–60.

52. Kiltz U, Essers I, Hiligsmann M, *et al*. "Which aspects of health are most important for patients with spondyloarthritis? A best worst scaling based on the ASAS Health Index" *Rheumatology*. 2016;55(10):1771–6. <https://doi.org/10.1093/rheumatology/kew238>.

53. Kiltz U, Baraliakos X, Karakostas P, *et al*. "Do patients with non-radiographic axial spondylarthritis differ from patients with ankylosing spondylitis?" *Arthritis Care Res*. 2012 Sep;64(9):1415–22. doi:10.1002/acr.21688. PMID: 22505331.

54. Kiltz U, van der Heijde D, Boonen A, *et al*. "Measuring impairments of functioning and health in patients with axial spondyloarthritis by using the ASAS Health Index and the Environmental Item Set: translation and cross-cultural adaptation into 15 languages" *RMD Open*. 2016 Oct 4;2(2):e000311. doi:10.1136/rmdopen-2016-000311. PMID: 27752358; PMCID: PMC5051462.

55. Kiltz U, Boonen A, van der Heijde D, *et al*. "Development of an environmental contextual factor item set relevant to global functioning and health in patients with axial spondyloarthritis" *Rheumatology*. 2021;keab653. <https://doi.org/10.1093/rheumatology/keab653>.

56. Kim JG, Jung J-Y, Lee J, *et al*. "Can whole spine magnetic resonance imaging predict radiographic progression and inflammatory activity in axial spondyloarthritis?" *Joint Bone Spine*, 2022:105352.

57. Kim J-W, Park S, Jung J-Y, *et al.* "Osteoporotic fracture in patients with ankylosing spondylitis: a multicenter comparative study of bone mineral density and the fracture risk assessment tool" *J Clin Med.* 2022;11:2830. https://doi.org/10.3390/jcm11102830

58. Koh TC. "Tai Chi and ankylosing spondylitis—A personal experience" *Am J Chinese Med.* 1982;10:59–61.

59. Lee T-H, Koo BS, Nam B, *et al.* "Age-stratified trends in the progression of spinal radiographic damage in patients with ankylosing spondylitis: a longitudinal study" *Ther Adv Musculoskel Dis.* 2022;14:1–12. doi:10.1177/1759720X221100301

60. Li Z, Khan MK, van der Linden S, et al. HLA-B27, axial spondyloarthritis, and survival. 2022 (submitted for publication).

61. Lim D, James N, Sobia H, *et al.* "Arthritis associated with acne conglobata, hidradenitis suppurativa and dissecting cellulitis of the scalp: A review with illustrative cases" *Curr Rheumatol Rep.* 2013 Aug;15(8):346. doi:10.1007/s11926-013-0346-y.

62. López-Medina C, Castro-Villegas MC, and Collantes-Estévez E. "Hip and shoulder involvement and their management in axial spondyloarthritis: a current review" *Curr Rheumatol Rep.* 2020;22:53. <https://doi.org/10.1007/s11926-020-00930-7>.

63. Mader R, Pappone N, Baraliakos X, *et al.* "Diffuse Idiopathic Skeletal Hyperostosis (DISH) and a possible inflammatory component" *Curr Rheumatol Rep.* 2021;23;6. <https://doi.org/10.1007/s11926-020-00972-x>.

64. Magrey MN, Danve AS, Ermann J, *et al.* "Recognizing axial spondyloarthritis: A guide for primary care" *Mayo Clin Proc.* 2020 Nov;95(11):2499–508. doi:10.1016/j.mayocp.2020.02.007. Epub 2020 Jul 29. PMID: 32736944.

65. Magrey M and Khan MA. "New insights into SAPHO syndrome" *Curr Rheumatol Report.* 2009 Oct;11(5):329–33.

66. Magrey M and Khan MA. "The paradox of bone formation and bone loss in ankylosing spondylitis: Evolving new concepts of bone formation and future trends in management" *Curr Rheumatol Rep.* 2017 Apr;19(4):17. doi:10.1007/s11926-017-0644-x.

67. Magrey M, Lewis S, and Khan MA. "Utility of DXA scanning and risk factors for osteoporosis in ankylosing spondylitis—A prospective study" *Semin Arthritis Rheum.* 2016;46:88–94.

68. Magrey M, Charles T, and Khan MA. "Relationship between disease activity measures, functional status, and fibromyalgia symptom scale in ankylosing spondylitis: a cross-sectional study" *J Clin Rheumatol.* 2020 Jul 22. doi:10.1097/RHU.0000000000001490.

69. Mandi P, Navarro-Compan V, Terslev L, *et al.* "EULAR recommendations for the use of imaging in diagnosis and management of spondyloarthritis in clinical practice" *Ann Rheum Dis.* 2015 Jul;74(7):1327–39. doi:10.1136/annrheumdis-2014-206971. Epub 2015 Apr 2.

70. Mauro D, Thomas R, Guggino G, *et al.* "Ankylosing spondylitis: An autoimmune or autoinflammatory disease?" *Nat Rev Rheumatol.* 2021;17:387–404. <https://doi.org/10.1038/s41584-021-00625-y>.

71. McHugh J. "Polygenic risk scores outperform other tests in AS" *Nat Rev Rheumatol* 2021;17:312. <https://doi.org/10.1038/s41584-021-00630-1>.

72. Mauro D, Thomas R, Guggino G, *et al.* "Ankylosing spondylitis: an autoimmune or autoinflammatory disease?" *Nat Rev Rheumatol.* 2021;17(7):387–404. doi:10.1038/s41584-021-00625-y

73. Mease P and Deodhar A. "Differentiating nonradiographic axial spondyloarthritis from its mimics: a narrative review" *BMC Musculoskelet Disord.* 2022;23(240). <https://doi.org/10.1186/s12891-022-05073-7>.

74. Michielsens CAJ, Broeder BD, Mulder MLM, *et al.* "Tumour necrosis factor inhibitor dose adaptation in psoriatic arthritis and axial spondyloarthritis (TAPAS): a retrospective cohort study" *Rheumatology.* 2022; 61(6):2307–2315. https://doi.org/10.1093/rheumatology/keab741

75. Mustafa KN, Hammoudeh M, and Khan MA. "HLA-B27 prevalence in Arab populations and among patients with ankylosing spondylitis" *J Rheumatol.* 2012 Aug;39(8):1675–7.

76. Navarro-Compan V, Sepriano A, El-Zorkani B, *et al.* "Axial spondyloarthritis" *Ann Rheum Dis.* 2021. doi:10.1136/annrheumdis-2021-221035.

77. Nikiphorou E, Santos EJF, Marques A, *et al.* "2021 EULAR recommendations for the implementation of self-management strategies in patients with inflammatory arthritis" *Ann Rheum Dis.* 2021. doi:10.1136/annrheumdis-2021-220249.

78. Nurmohamed M, Heslinga M, and Kitas G. "Cardiovascular comorbidity in rheumatic diseases" *Nat Rev Rheumatol.* 2015;11:693–704. <https://doi.org/10.1038/nrrheum.2015.112>.

79. Olivieri I, D'Angelo S, Palazzi P, *et al.* "Diffuse Idiopathic Skeletal Hyperostosis: A condition that needs to be differentiated from spondyloarthritis" *Curr Rheumatol Report.* 2009 Oct;11(5):321–8.

80. Olivieri I, D'Angelo S, Cutro MS, *et al.* "Diffuse Idiopathic Skeletal Hyperostosis may give the typical postural abnormalities of advanced ankylosing spondylitis" *Rheumatol.* (Oxford). 2007;46(11):1709–11.

81. Ostensen M and Ostensen H. "Ankylosing spondylitis—The female aspect" *J Rheumatol.* 1998;25:120–4.

82. Ozgocmen S, Akgul O, and Khan MA. "Mnemonic for assessment of the spondyloarthritis international society criteria" *J Rheumatol.* 2010 Sep;37(9):1978.

83. Ozgocmen S and Khan MA. "Current concept of spondyloarthritis: Special emphasis on early referral and diagnosis" *Curr Rheumatol Report.* 2012 Oct;14(5):409–14. doi:10.1007/s11926-012-0274-2. Erratum: 2012 Dec;14(6):624. doi:10.1007/s11926-012-0274-2.

84. Pincus T, Bergman MJ, and Yazici Y. "RAPID3-an index of physical function, pain, and global status as 'vital signs' to improve care for people with chronic rheumatic diseases" *Bull NYU Hosp Jt Dis.* 2009;67(2):211–25.

85. Poddubnyy D, Weineck H, Diekhoff T, *et al.* "Clinical and imaging characteristics of osteitis condensans ilii as compared with axial spondyloarthritis" *Rheumatology.* 2020 Dec;59(12):3798–806.

86. Poddubnyy D. "Classification vs diagnostic criteria: the challenge of diagnosing axial spondyloarthritis" *Rheumatology.* 2020 Oct;59(4):iv6–iv17. <https://doi.org/10.1093/rheumatology/keaa250>.

87. Qaiyum Z, Lim M, Inman RD. "The gut–joint axis in spondyloarthritis: immunological, microbial, and clinical insights" *Semin Immunopathol.* 2021 Apr;43(2):173–92. doi:10.1007/s00281-021-00845-0. Epub 2021 Feb 24. PMID: 33625549.

88. Raja SN, Carr DB, Cohen M, *et al.* "The revised International Association for the Study of Pain definition of pain: concepts, challenges, and compromises" *Pain.* 2020 Sep 1;161(9):1976–82. doi:10.1097/j.pain.0000000000001939.

89. Rajkomar A, Dean J and Kohane I. Machine learning in medicine, New England J Med. 2019 Apr 4;380(14):1347–58.

90. Ranganathan V, Gracey E, Brown M, *et al.* "Pathogenesis of ankylosing spondylitis—recent advances and future directions" *Nat Rev Rheumatol.* 2017;13:359–67. <https://doi.org/10.1038/nrrheum.2017.56>.

91. Ritchlin C and Adamopoulos IE. "Axial spondyloarthritis: New advances in diagnosis and management" *BMJ.* 2021 Jan 4;372:m4447. doi:10.1136/bmj.m4447. PMID: 33397652.

92. Robinson PC, van der Linden S, Khan MA, *et al.* "Axial spondyloarthritis: Concept, construct, classification, and implications for therapy" *Nat Rev Rheumatol.* 2021. <https://doi.org/10.1038/s41584-020-00552-4>.

93. Rosenbaum JT, Hamilton H, Weisman M, *et al.* "The effect of HLA-B27 0n susceptibility and severity of COVID-19" *Rheumatol.* 2021 Apr;48(4):621–2.

94. Rudwaleit M, Khan MA, and Sieper J. "The challenge of diagnosis and classification in early ankylosing spondylitis: Do we need new criteria?" *Arthritis Rheum.* 2005;52:1000–8.

95. Rudwaleit M, van der Heijde D, Khan MA, *et al.* "How to diagnose axial spondyloarthropathy early?" *Ann Rheum Dis* 2004;63:535–43.

96. Rudwaleit M, van der Heijde D, Landewé R, *et al.* "The development of Assessment in SpondyloArthritis International Society (ASAS) classification criteria for axial spondyloarthritis (Part II): Validation and final selection" *Ann Rheum Dis.* 2009;68(6):777–83.

97. Rueda-Gotor H, Ferraz-Amaro I, Genre F, *et al.* "Factors associated with atherosclerosis in radiographic and non-radiographic axial spondyloarthritis. A multicenter study on 838 patients" *Semin Arthritis Rheum.* 2022;Vil 55:152037.

98. Sharma M, Jain N, Wang D, *et al.* "Impact of age on mortality and complications in patients with ankylosing spondylitis spine fractures" *J Clin Neuroscience.* 2021;85:188–97.

99. Shresthaa S, Brand JS, Järåse J, *et al.* "Association between inflammatory bowel disease and spondyloarthritis: findings from a nationwide study in Sweden" *J Crohn's Colitis.* Published: 05 May 2022. doi:10.1093/ecco-jcc/jjac065

100. Sieper J and Poddubnyy D. "Axial spondyloarthritis" *Lancet.* 2017 Jul 1;390(10089):73–84.

101. Sieper J, Rudwaleit M, Khan MA, *et al.* "Concept and epidemiology of spondyloarthritis" *Best Pract Res Clin Rheumatol.* 2006;23(3):401–17.

102. Sieper J, van der Heijde D, Landewé R, *et al.* "New criteria for inflammatory back pain in patients with chronic back pain—A real patient exercise of the Assessment in SpondyloArthritis International Society (ASAS)" *Ann Rheum Dis.* 2009

103. Sieper J, Poddubnyy D, and Miossec P. "The IL-23–IL-17 pathway as a therapeutic target in axial spondyloarthritis" *Nat Rev Rheumatol.* 2019 Dec;15(12):747–57.

104. Srinivasalu H, Treemarcki EB, and Redmond C. "Advances in juvenile spondyloarthritis" *Curr Rheumatol Rep.* 2021 Jul 13;23(9):70. PubMed PMID: 34255209.

105. Taams LS, Steel KJA, Srenathan U, *et al.* "IL-17 in the immunopathogenesis of spondyloarthritis" *Nat Rev Rheumatol.* 2018;14:453–66. doi:10.1038/s41584-018-0044-2.

106. Tanaka Y, Luo Y, O'Shea JJ, *et al.* "Janus kinase-targeting therapies in rheumatology: A mechanisms-based approach" *Nat Rev Rheumatol.* 2022 Jan 5:1–13. doi:10.1038/s41584-021-00726-8.

107. van der Heijde D, Daikh DI, Betteridge N, *et al.* "Common language description of the term rheumatic and musculoskeletal diseases (RMDs) for use in communication with the lay public, healthcare providers and other stakeholders endorsed by the European League Against Rheumatism (EULAR) and the American College of Rheumatology (ACR)" *Ann Rheum Dis.* 2018;77:829–32.

108. van der Linden SM, Valkenburg HA, Cats A. Evaluation of diagnostic criteria for ankylosing spondylitis. A proposal for modification of the new york criteria. *Arthritis Rheum.* 1984;27:361–8.

109. van der Linden SM, Valkenberg HA, de Jongh B, *et al.* "The risk of developing ankylosing spondylitis in HLA-B27 positive individuals. A comparison of relatives of spondylitis patients with the general population" *Arthritis Rheum.* 1984;27:241–9.

110. van der Linden SM, Khan MA, Li Z, *et al.* "Factors predicting axial spondlyoarthritis among first-degree relatives of probands with ankylosing spondylitis. A family study spanning 35 years" *Ann Rheum Dis.* 2022 Mar. <http://dx.doi.org/10.1136/annrheumdis-2021-222083>.

111. van der Linden SM, Khan MA, Li Z, *et al.* Recurrence of axial spondyloarthritis among first-degree relatives in a prospective 35-year-followup family study. *RMD Open.* 2022;8:e002208. doi:10.1136/rmdopen-2022-002208

112. Weber U, Pfirrmann CWA, Kissling RO, *et al.* "Early spondyloarthritis in HLA-B27 positive monozygotic twin pair: A highly concordant onset, sites of involvement, and disease course" *J Rheumatol.* 2008;35(7):1464–7.

113. Weber U, *et al*. "Imaging in axial spondyloarthritis: What is relevant for diagnosis in daily practice" *Curr Rheumatol Rep.* 2021 Jul 3;23(8):66. PubMed PMID: 34218356.

114. Wendling D, Hecquet S, Fogel O, *et al.* "2022 French Society for Rheumatology (SFR) recommendations on the everyday management of patients with spondyloarthritis, including psoriatic arthritis" *Joint Bone Spine.* 2022. <https://doi.org/10.1016/j.jbspin.2022.105344>.

115. Wetterslev M, Georgiadis S, Sørensen IJ, *et al.* "Tapering of TNF inhibitors in axial spondyloarthritis in routine care—2-year clinical and MRI outcomes and predictors of successful tapering" *Rheumatology.* 2021:keab755. <https://doi.org/10.1093/rheumatology/keab755>.

116. Winthrop KL, Nash P, Yamaoka K, *et al.* "Incidence and risk factors for herpes zoster in patients with rheumatoid arthritis receiving upadacitinib: a pooled analysis of six phase III clinical trials" *Ann Rheum Dis.* doi:10.1136/annrheumdis-2021-220822.

117. Xie Y, Xu E, Bowe B, *et al.* "Long term cardiovascular outcomes of COVID-19" *Nat Med.* 2022;28:583.

118. Yagan R and Khan MA. "Confusion of roentgenographic differential diagnosis between ankylosing hyperostosis (Forestier's disease) and ankylosing spondylitis" *Clin Rheumatol.* 1983;2:285–92.

119. Zaarour N, Li Y, Shi H, *et al.* "From the genetics of ankylosing spondylitis to new biology and drug target discovery" *Front Immunol.* 2021 Feb 17. <https://doi.org/10.3389/fimmu.2021.624632>.

120. Zhang Y and Wang C. "Acupuncture and chronic musculoskeletal pain" *Curr Rheumatol Rep.* 2020;22:80. <https://doi.org/10.1007/s11926-020-00954-z>.

121. Zhang S, Peng L, Li Q, *et al.* "Spectrum of spondyloarthritis among Chinese populations" *Curr Rheumatol Rep.* 2022;24:247=258. <https://doi.org/10.1007/s11926-022-01079-1>.

122. Zhao SS, Pittman B, Harrison NL, *et al.* "Diagnostic delay in axial spondyloarthritis: A systemic review and meta-analysis" *Rheumatology.* 2021;60(4):1620–8.

Index